HARVEST OF HOPE

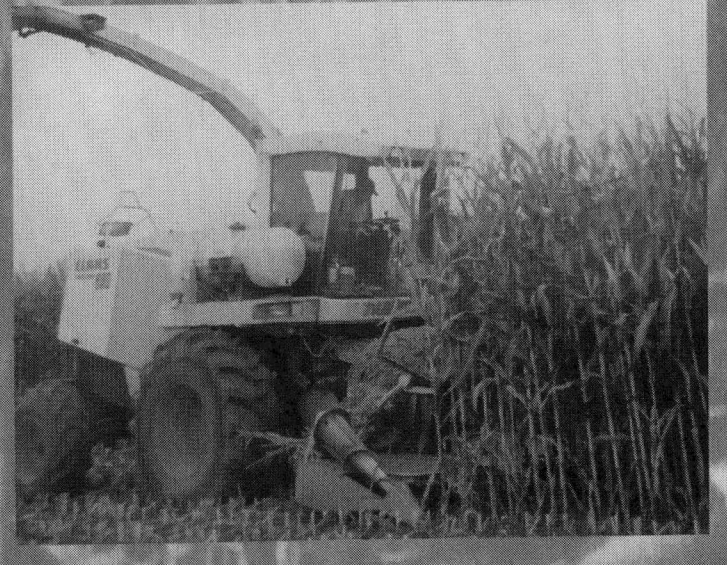

Conquering Brain CANCER

BARBARA RAMSEY

2

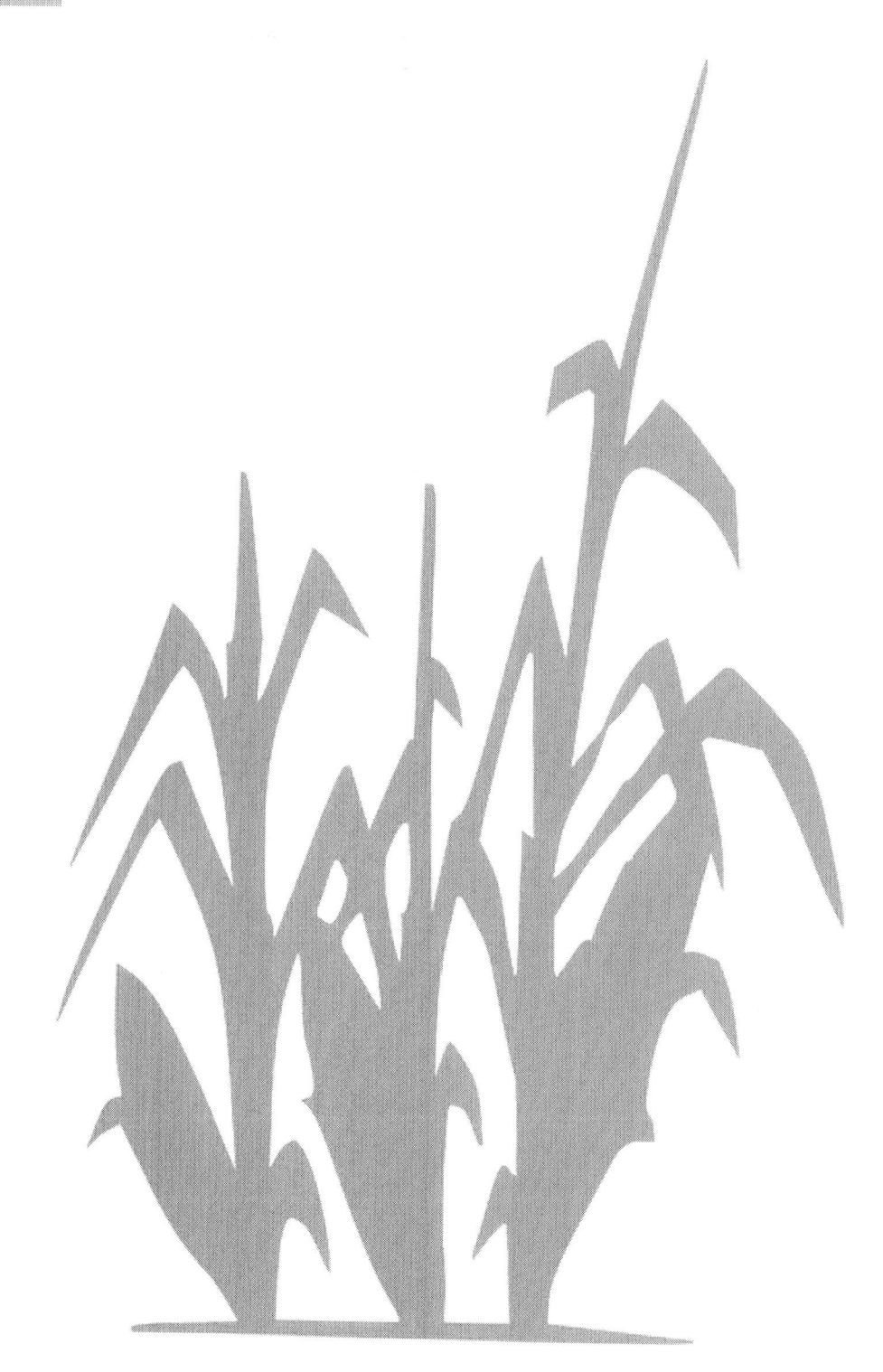

HARVEST OF HOPE

Conquering Brain Cancer

BARBARA RAMSEY

© 2019 Barbara Ramsey

HARVEST OF HOPE by Barbara Ramsey

Cover Design by Ann Miesner

Printed in the United States of America

ISBN: 978-1090335135

All rights are reserved solely by the author. The author guarantees all contents are original and do not infringe upon the legal rights of any other person or work. No part of this book may be reproduced in any form without the permission of the author at: bramsey0208@gmail.com.

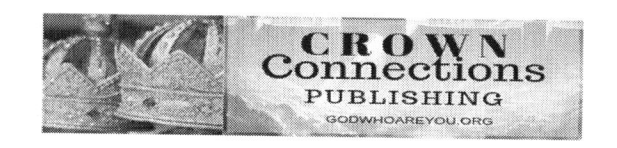

CROWN Connections PUBLISHING
GODWHOAREYOU.ORG

DEDICATION

To Amy Slade

You listened to me, a new widow, over the course of several weeks, voice out loud the true account of the fresh, painful, yet miraculous experience I had just lived through. By the time I finished, we had become genuine friends in all the ways that mattered. You implanted within me the vision that writing my story could inspire others who might be going through a similar valley in their lives, to reach up for help and hope through faith. Without your continuing encouragement along this journey, this book might never have reached completion.

Thank you,
Amy, my forever 'soul sister.'

6

TABLE OF CONTENTS

1. The Waiting Game: June 10, 2010..................9
2. The Milestone: 2 Days Earlier..................12
3. The Two Shall Become One: 7 Months Earlier, October, 2009..................15
4. The Pain Breaker: The Next Day..................25
5. The Little Morphine Men..................31
6. The Revelation: Late November, 2009..................37
7. The Kodak Moment..................48
8. Badminton, Anyone? January, 2010..................52
9. The Unfortunate Moment in Time: June 10, 2010..................61
10. The Moment of Truth: June 14, 2010..................72
11. The Referral: Several Days Later..................79
12. The Season of Miracles: June 29, 2010..................88
13. The Painful Thorn..................93
14. The Unexpected Helper: Early July, 2010......110
15. The Treatment Journey: Late July, 2010.........116

16. The Guardian Angel: August 25, 2010............126
17. The Day of Decision: The Next Day...............137
18. The Graduation: Late September, 2010..........144
19. The Homecoming...152
20. The Last Harvest: October, 2010.....................156
21. The Sad Good-bye: November, 2010..............163
22. The Love of Family...170
23. The Great Reveal: Spring, 2011......................177
24. The Cruise into Transition:
    April, 2011...183
25. The Second Haven: Late April, 2011..............195
26. The Mysterious Walk: May, 2011......................206
27. The Healing: Late June, 2011............................215

What Cancer Cannot Do..225

Chapter 1
The Waiting Game

June 10, 2010

THE SURREAL BLUE LIGHTING and the eerie silence at the nurses' station. That is the strongest memory incapsulating the twenty-five minutes that changed our lives forever.

We had been patiently, then impatiently, waiting for over four solid hours for the doctor to make his appearance in the neurological unit on the fifth floor of the Albuquerque hospital. We had been here for two excruciatingly long days.

"The doctor usually makes his rounds about five or five-thirty," the nurse assured us. I had also asked another nurse and a couple of aides during the long afternoon. I had found it was wise to take the average of several opinions to arrive at a correct answer in the typical realm of timing in the medical world.

When the dinner tray arrived a little after 5:30 p.m., we were temporarily distracted from our clock-watching. Jim's appetite was better, finally, and his strange symptoms had altogether subsided. He was chomping at the bits to get out of that hospital and back to the farm, where the hay fields were waiting to be relieved of the heavy rows of newly-raked alfalfa.

My mind wandered back to those familiar hay circles that we had come to know intimately over the past ten years since we had made the life-changing decision for Jim to take the job of farm manager on a huge farm in New Mexico. It was a long distance from our last home back in western Kansas, where we had lived and worked for over seventeen years. Our children had grown up there. All three boys had graduated from high school there. We were now empty nesters and had taken this job far away from our family in order to become debt-free. We quickly fell in love with the arid desert climate and the wonderful people we met. I thought about this farm we had come to know so well.

I could smell the fresh scent of bright-green alfalfa laying in neat paths of diminishing circles. The pattern resembled a dart board after I had cut the one hundred-twenty-acre fields with the gigantic thirty-foot green swather. I could see the headlights of the tractors pulling the noisy clanking balers as they hungrily ate up the strips of hay, spitting out huge, neatly-compacted, wrapped square bales every few yards under a night sky brilliantly lit with a vast array of shimmering stars. I could see the piles of various sizes of stones stacked in the corners of some of the rockier fields. They represented long tedious days of sore backs and sunbaked skin and tired muscles. We had hand-picked the rocks day after day the first spring we moved onto the farm.

I thought about the individual cantankerous quirks of each of the electric irrigation systems that traveled slowly around the field from a pivot motor in the center of each of the twenty-five circles of cropland. They watered every inch of those thirsty corn and alfalfa and triticale plants during eight tedious months of each year.

Jim knew every single farm trail that led in and out and around each of those giant circles of crops. He knew every shortcut of the route to arrive at the exact spot where he wanted to hand-check the moisture in a particular row. From years of experience, he knew precisely when it was time to call out the baler operators to begin the arduous task of bringing the crops to completion under the hay sheds for their final place of rest.

He could find his way on cloudy moonless nights. He could maneuver those trails on pitch-dark nights with the only lights coming from the high beams of his farm truck headlights. I often marveled at the effortless automatic skill he displayed as I would sit in the passenger seat and observe him on unconscious autopilot. He slowed down for the sandy spot and swerved just in time to miss the mud hole. He could be studying the tiniest detail of the crops and dodge a stray rock that had worked its way to the surface of the road without even thinking about it. He literally had memorized every square inch of those three thousand acres, and it had become his domain.

Chapter 2
The Milestone

2 Days Earlier

HE WALKED IN THE FRONT DOOR of our farmhouse visibly shaken! Suppertime had long since passed, the kitchen was clean, and I was just out of the hot shower. I was thinking of those cool fresh sheets on the bed and how good it would feel to stretch my weary body upon them. I looked up to find confusion and fear written all over the face of my usually confident husband.

"I couldn't find the field," he softly spoke, concern and pain betraying his calmness.

"What do you mean, Jim?"

I became aware that a lengthy amount of time had passed since he had left the house earlier to "run out and check a couple of hay fields." But I had learned long ago as a farmer's wife that at this time of year there were multiple tasks going on all over the farm, and Jim was responsible to oversee them all. Long hours of labor continued at all hours of night and day, and it was routine for a problem to arise at any given location around the huge acreage.

This had been our way of life for most all the forty years of our marriage, and it didn't appear that it would be any different for at least another good ten years. Early retirement and leisurely travel were not in our plans, and we had accepted this reality long ago. Jim was a farmer, through and through. We had always worked hard for every cent we got and didn't expect a free ride ahead as long as we could put both feet on the floor every morning.

"I was driving out to check the moisture on Circle 17, and everything became muddled in my mind. I drove around and nothing looked familiar to me. Finally, I saw the bright lights from the dairy and started driving toward them. I stopped and sat there in the pickup for a long time until finally it all came back into focus. I knew where I was. I drove right over to 17 and the hay was dry enough to call out the balers . . . ." He turned and slowly trudged toward the bedroom, leaving me stunned and spinning with unanswered questions.

"Did you bump your head on anything earlier today? Is your eyesight okay? Do you have a headache? How long were you like this?" I wanted it to make sense, to figure it all out so I could fix the problem and never have to see that look of helpless confusion on my husband's face ever again.

"Barb, I'm tired and just want to go to bed."

I heard the shower start and the bathroom door slide shut. I knew he was through talking, and I immediately turned my fears toward the Lord.

"Dear God, please be with my husband tonight. If he is just overly tired, Lord, give him a restful night of sleep. Whatever might have caused this confusion, please take it away and allow him to wake up refreshed and clear-minded. Thank you for your faithfulness in always taking care of us. In Jesus name, Amen."

As I lay there still and waiting in the cool calmness of night, with the shower pattering soothing drops of water on my husband's weary body, my mind went back seven months to the other 'strange episode.' Although it was scary and beyond stressful, we thought the final diagnosis had solved the big mystery of severe symptoms that had come on with a vengeance and wracked Jim's body with unrelenting pain for five long days.

Chapter 3
The Two Shall Become One

7 Months Earlier

THE INCIDENT HAD STARTED with a headache that wouldn't respond to any normal solution. Jim had tried all the variety of over-the-counter pain and headache relievers to no avail. After lunch, he had stayed home for an extra hour with his eyes closed and his head laid back in his recliner. After a call from one of the workers, he was out the door again to solve one of the dozen situations which arise on a busy farm every day.

I could tell the pain was great, but this was one tough man to bring down. I had seen him work right through bouts of flu, a back out of place, kidney-stone attacks, and other miscellaneous illnesses. He lived by the unwritten law: you can't keep a good man down. I called our local hometown's physician assistant (PA), leaving a voice message asking if I should bring my stubborn husband in to be checked over. A couple of hours later, the return call from Dr. Susan concerned me a little:

"Persistent headaches are nothing to mess around with. I could check him out here, but if the pain continues to be as strong as you are describing, I would advise you take him into Albuquerque to run him through some tests."

A very pale and unsteady husband came back in the door late in the afternoon. The pain was worse, and he had thrown up. I was ready to go the seventy miles into the city. We needed to leave right away. All the hesitancy or doubt had been used up, absorbed completely by common sense and logic. Something was wrong and we had to find out what it was. This was not one of those times when it would just all go away. I began to feel the dread wash over me as we began the hour and ten-minute drive that drug out much too long.

"Pull over, Barb!"

"I can't right here, but I will as soon as I get around this curve." We were right in the middle of rush hour traffic, going through the many curves descending further into the mountains as we headed into the big valley that is Albuquerque.

"Pull over right here! I can't wait."

I pulled over, and Jim's head was immediately out of the car. I hurt for him as he held his aching head. After almost forty years of being married to the same person, I honestly COULD feel his pain. My hands were shaking as I pulled back into the heavy traffic. I kept telling myself to be calm. This was one of those times when I longed for the nearness of family—at least one single person to share the burden with.

But even better, I had the Lord to stand with us every moment. He knew every detail about what was ahead of us. Little did I understand at this very abrupt, intrusive moment into our relatively normal lives, even a tiny fraction of what lay ahead. And what it means to really trust.

Hours and hours later, I sat in the straight chair next to the hospital bed where my husband lay hooked up to the IV dripping fluids into his six-foot-two-inch body. After stopping off at an urgent-care facility on the east side of town, the doctor on staff sent us quickly on our way to the nearest hospital emergency room. Any hope of a quick fix to Jim's pain was dimming swiftly. After a brief physical exam and a list of verbal questions, he had summed up his take on the matter with just a few words:

"When you are dealing with head pain this severe not due to trauma, the only way to find out what is causing it is to run a series of tests including an MRI, CT Scan, etc. I will call ahead to let them know you are on the way."

A few blocks west, we pulled into the emergency room parking lot of the nearest hospital. By this time, my heart was racing, and we began to realize that this was going to be a very long night. I anticipated hours of waiting in the ER holding area. This fact was not based on pessimism, but actual experience. One night we had waited all night just to be seen for one of Jim's kidney-stone episodes. The stone passed on its own before we even got called back to an exam room; not so surprising considering about eight tedious hours had gone by.

The fact this didn't occur now brought even more soberness to the situation at hand. Even the paperwork was postponed, with the nurses only asking a few minimal questions while they whisked us through to the first of many medical procedures to follow. During all this time, Jim's pain throbbed on. The pain issue had finally been addressed with a shot of morphine into the IV. Surprisingly, it produced little relief.

We moved from one area of the hospital to the other as each test was administered. In the radiology department, a dye was injected into the body for the Contrast MRI. The test required him to lie completely still while the machine scanned the entire head, producing detailed images using magnets, radio waves, and a computer.

Each procedure was long and tedious. I knew Jim was exhausted, and a heavy weight of fatigue settled over my entire body as the hours wore on. No use to call and wake anyone up at this time of night, as I had nothing conclusive to tell. I would wait until morning to let a few close friends and family know. When we left home late in the afternoon, I had called to start a prayer chain going for us. I knew these friends of ours would earnestly pray us through this ordeal.

"Lord, we are in your hands. I feel so all alone in the middle of the night in a big hospital I am not in the least familiar with. Give us strength and patience. Most of all, give Jim relief from this tremendous pain. Help the doctors to have wisdom to know what is causing this and give them knowledge to know what to do. I know you are in control of all of this. You are bigger than any problem we might face. In Jesus name, AMEN."

Trust and faith and hope. We had lived by these three words for many years. We wouldn't stop now.

The tests were over; the pain remained; the endless night drug on. Finally, officially admitted, I glanced in the bathroom mirror in Jim's hospital room. Shocked, I looked closer. Disheveled hair, make-up long gone from the many tears shed, clothes wrinkled. All understood. But why was I so PALE? I glanced back at Jim's pain-wracked face and saw the same look reflected in the mirror: "The two shall become one."

I heard the bed rolling down the hallway toward our room. Thank God for small favors! When the male nurse had taken Jim's vitals last time, I pleaded with him for a small cot, a recliner, or just anything better than two hard, straight-backed chairs placed front-to-front. Oh, and one small pillow. No blanket. And NO way of getting any rest or comfort.

"We live seventy miles from here, and I can't go home. We have been up all night going through this. There is no other patient in the room. Would you please see what you can do?"

I saw compassion in the young man's eyes. I also saw doubt. But he agreed to try.

The wheels of the cot stopped maybe two doors from our room. "Where are you going with that bed?" a sharp demanding voice asked.

"To room 204. The new admit. They live a long way out of town and the wife has asked for a bed."

"It is a two-patient room and we cannot put a cot in there!"

"But it is 3:00 a.m."

"Take the bed back!"

The wheels started rolling again, but I couldn't believe my ears. It was going back from where it came! I popped up off the chair with a renewed burst of adrenaline. The young nurse stuck his head in the door.

"I'm sorry, but my supervisor told me we can't have another bed in here."

I wanted to scream at him, go out in the hall and scream at his supervisor, *go out and wake somebody up and scream at them!*

Out of the darkness, Jim's weak voice sounded. "Come over here, honey, and crawl in bed with me."

The wind dropped quickly out of my sails. I could literally feel my body curled up next to my husband's always-warm one, where I could relax and just doze for a while. The exhaustion lured me toward the bed. But just as everything was abnormal during this ordeal, even the natural simple act of lying cuddled up beside my husband was not possible.

"No, honey, I can't. There's not enough room, and it would make you even more uncomfortable."

I knew Jim had not had a wink of sleep either. Although he was at least reclining, his big frame hung over the end of the short bed about two inches, and the headache persisted with a vengeance. The button strapped around his wrist enabled him to give himself a boost of morphine when he felt the need, but the amount was still controlled. So far, at best, it had only dulled the pain for a short time.

I returned to the hard chair. This endless night would eventually be over. I remembered the promise Jim and I had made to each other years before. If one of us was in the hospital, the other one would stay in the room and make sure the care was given, no mistakes occurred with medicines and procedures, and we would be each other's adversary. No matter how long the stay was. No matter how hard the chairs were.

The breakfast tray finally rolled into the room. I stiffly scooted back the second chair, making room for the tray to be rolled up close to the hospital bed. It was a maneuver I had gotten quite adept at during the long, night hours as the parade of nurses and aides came in and out to perform their assigned duties. The light would flip on, a variety of voices would ask,

"Mr. McCune? Please give me your date of birth. I am here to take your vitals, or check your IV, or draw some blood."

Numbness crept upon my brain as the adrenaline of the previous day had gradually faded to a dull game of waiting. *What would the results of the many tests tell us? When would the doctor make his rounds? How long would we have to stay here? When would Jim's pain ever stop?* These questions became the focus. *Since it was now daylight, should I start making phone calls to relatives and friends? What could I even tell them?*

Vitals throughout the night were consistent. Blood pressure: running high, which was normal with the amount of pain; Pulse: normal; Temperature: normal; Oxygen level: low. This was puzzling and had been stabilized with oxygen added to the other equipment dangling from my husband's body.

While the clock continued to tick on, I walked out into the hall to call the farm shop. The workers would be arriving and needed direction for the day's tasks. As always, Jim had already been stewing over his inability to be present in body and had given me specific instructions to pass on. All the guys had a highly respectful relationship with their boss.

Over the last few years, a strong team had formed. Although this had taken a while to create, we now cared about and were personally involved in each one of our expanded farm family. Unlike many workers we had previously encountered, who only cared about collecting the paycheck, these men worked diligently toward getting the crops in and staying with the task until it was successfully completed. That attitude had made our lives much easier, and we were faithful to thank God for this extra blessing of unity.

As I was walking and talking on the cell phone, two very welcome faces rounded the nurses' desk. As I closed the phone, I sank into their welcome hugs with relief. Here were two people we had come to love dearly in our time in New Mexico. Don was our enthusiastic Sunday school teacher and Bible study leader, and Carita's caring heart and loving spirit had filled so many needs in our lives over the span of time we had gotten to know them well.

"Barb! We have been praying faithfully for you and Jim all night long off and on. What have you found out, and is there anything we can do?"

Tears began running freely down my cheeks. They led me over to the couches in the middle of the open waiting area. What a comfort to be in the presence of such caring friends! I poured out the events of the previous day and expressed my deep concern that nothing had yet fazed the persistent headache.

A doctor strode briskly up to the nurses' station and began shuffling through the patient files. Hopefully, this would be the man who could give us some answers. My friends urged me to go ahead and return to Jim's room. They would be back again later to check on us. Taking a deep breath, I followed the doctor into Jim's room where the breakfast tray lay untouched.

Flipping through Jim's chart, the doctor peered over his squared glasses. "It appears nothing serious has shown up from all the procedures. The only disturbance is a slight bleed appearing on the MRI, probably the result of a small broken artery or vein; but not a continuous bleed situation. Probably a singular incident caused by pressure in the brain, maybe from the headache. The only other abnormality is the low oxygen level."

"Then what is causing the pain?"

"I will be consulting with a neurologist about this issue today and will see you again this evening. We'll observe how you get along in the next few hours."

Not a very conclusive observation. There was too much puzzlement in his demeanor. I sensed he didn't know what to tell us. He simply walked out the door and proceeded on to the next patient––leaving us in limbo.

I was beyond exhaustion. Stress can take its toll so quickly, especially after a lost night of sleep. No make-up or comb or fresh clothes. I had brushed my teeth with the kit of necessities brought by for Jim. By this time, I had no shame. When Jim scooted over and once again motioned for me to come lie down beside him, I carefully crawled in amongst the tangle of cords and pulled up the side rail so I wouldn't fall off the narrow bed. Oh, the sweet relief of relaxation, if only for a few precious moments!

Turned away from Jim, once again tears slid down my face as he tightened up once more in pain and softly groaned. I felt him push the button again, and he wrapped his arm around me tightly.

"It's going to be okay," I assured him brightly. Thank goodness he couldn't see my face.

"God will take care of us as He always has." This I could say with assurance. I drifted off for some sweet escape.

"Oh, don't get up!" I jumped at the sound of a woman's voice in the room. "My name is Mary Scott, and I am in charge of patient advocacy. Is there anything I can do for you?"

She shouldn't have asked if she didn't want an earful. I quietly slid down the bars and walked toward the door, closing it softly behind us. I quickly recapped the experience of the previous night, simply sticking to the facts. No one else had been admitted and assigned to share our room.

With kindness in her eyes, she handed me her card and jotted down a few notes to herself. She handed me a form and explained that if I would write down what I had just told her, she would make sure the matter was swiftly addressed. After apologizing profusely, she also reassured me that I would not spend another night there without a bed to sleep in.

To my surprise, that night we actually slept in a motel room across town. Later in the afternoon, the doctor reappeared with a plan of action. "I have spoken with a neurologist and she can see you tomorrow. Perhaps she will be able to figure out the source of your pain."

I appreciated a plan of action instead of stalling us out in the hospital for another night without any change. The only apprehension I had was what to do with a husband still in such a state of great pain. I was thinking it would not be a good idea to take him all the way back home seventy miles away from hospital facilities. *What would we do if he started vomiting again or something else burst in his head?*

"I will give you a strong prescription for pain that should get him through the night."

Still not practical, I was thinking. I had seen how many times Jim had punched the morphine button.

It was pitch dark by the time we were finally released to find a motel. It would have been hours earlier, except for one pesky problem. Before Jim could pass the release, he had to show stable vitals. Numbers had to be within a certain range. Everything else stabilized except for the oxygen level. Once the machine was taken off, the level would take a nosedive. He finally passed the test by taking a series of very deep breaths. I was not very encouraged, and it niggled at my brain. But this issue was not my biggest worry now. We were out in the dark and it was totally up to me to find a place for us to stay.

I had gotten familiar enough with Albuquerque over the past few years, but my vision at night was not the best, and my brain was now numb. In the daytime it is easy to keep your bearings. Just look for the mountains and you will know where you are. That theory doesn't work at night. Plus, I had to find an open pharmacy and fill the pain prescription.

Jim had always been the one with the good sense of direction. When I seemed hesitant, he tried to guide me across town. Often coming to the city for farm parts, he knew street names and areas of town I didn't; however, this time he couldn't remember names or get himself oriented. If I had taken in as much morphine as he had over the last twenty-four hours, I wouldn't even have known my own name, much less the street names.

Again, I began to pray: "Lord help me find these places I need to go. And please help us find a room at the first place we stop."

An hour later, we were safely in a nice motel. Although I wouldn't have cared how much the room cost, I was thankful when the clerk told me there was a reduced rate for medical reasons, and they were running a special. *When was the last time I had eaten?*

All I longed for was a good shower and a soft bed, and especially a safe and restful night for Jim. He looked awful. So did I. I lay in the dark room and thanked God for the stillness, the cleanliness, and the privacy. The respite before the next wave washed over us.

Chapter 4

The Pain Breaker

The Next Day

WAS IT REALLY THURSDAY MORNING? We were sitting in the waiting room of the neurologist, and I was filling out the endless paper routine again. Our friend Gary was on the phone reminding Jim of the trip we were taking together out to Las Vegas for the National Drag Races. I had totally blocked that out of my mind, and it wasn't until I heard Jim tell Gary we were still going, that I zeroed in on what he was talking about. I motioned for Jim to let me talk to Gary.

As Jim handed me the phone, I whispered to him, "Honey, there is no way we will be able to go. We have to get this all figured out, and they are leaving in just a couple of days."

"You don't know that. I think I will be okay by then."

The pain meds were talking. I got on the phone, and briefly filled Gary in on the situation. Of course he understood and wished us the best.

"Let me know what you find out, and just take care of that Jim."

The receptionist called our name.

I wanted so badly for this doctor to figure it out. We were both desperate for the answer about the source of the headache. I recited the events over the last forty-eight hours in great detail. Jim was asked dozens of questions. This doctor was sincere and caring and intent on helping. She was an expert in this field. As she viewed the MRI disk, test results, and reviewed the notes from Jim's chart, I prayed silently. I kept glancing at the man I loved holding his head in his hands.

"Pressure causes pain. Infection causes pain. The only way to know is to knock out the possibilities one by one. The small bleed on the MRI does not warrant this type of pain. It could be a result of high blood pressure causing the vessel to break, but that does not explain the origin of the problem. After we determine this, then you need to come back and we will address the issue of the low oxygen. I would like for you to go through the sleep clinic.

"Apnea can cause a peak of high blood pressure followed by a diminished oxygen level. For now, I am going to call the main hospital downtown where they have a small neurology unit. I will get you in there this afternoon and ask one of the neurologists on staff to order some further testing. One of these will be a spinal tap which will test the pressure in the lining of the brain, making sure an infection hasn't settled in. This can be quite serious. I will fax my notes immediately to the hospital so you can be admitted right away."

I was impressed by the logic of her words and ready to proceed. *A possible infection in his brain? What would that mean?* I could see the concern in her face as she mentioned it.

If there was a neurology department in the downtown hospital, why didn't they tell us before admitting us to the smaller hospital a couple of nights ago? They were owned by the same medical network.

We could have been at least a day closer to an answer if they had just told us to drive there first. There was no use dwelling on it now. We walked slowly to the car arm in arm.

Amazingly, the admission process was pretty quick. It helped tremendously that the neurologist had called over to the hospital and cleared the paper maze path ahead for us. Thank God for large favors!

Upstairs, about forty-five minutes later, we were settled in a small private room in the neurology unit. I felt more secure, more hopeful this would be the place we would find answers. By this time, we had left a trail of paperwork a mile long behind us. When we first met the neurologist at this hospital, he had reviewed our story and personally talked to the other neurologist we had seen that morning. Our case was not the easy prognosis. I again sensed puzzlement and uncertainty.

About the only test left to do was the spinal tap. It was scheduled for the next day. My friend had connected with us again and brought by some basic necessities including a Bible. In the dim light of the cracked bathroom door, I read a few verses from Psalms out loud. Any bright light increased the pain for Jim, and I had folded out the vinyl chair into a straight cot-like bed in the faint light. Not very comfortable, but at least I could stretch out straight and have as many blankets as I wanted. Pillows, however, were a scarce commodity. Not one available in the whole huge hospital. Being the least of my worries, I requested another blanket and folded it up into a hard pillow.

By this time, Jim had become embroiled into a vicious circle of morphine and endless pain. The one bright spot occurred when a kind nurse brought in a heated blanket straight from the dryer for him. Those are the small miracles in a time of tangled webs of fatigue and question marks. I remember falling to sleep thinking how it was time for me to be the strong one—to take over the responsibility of asking the right questions and making sure my husband was taken care of.

"Help me Lord, to find the strength."

Standing in the bathroom the next morning in the cold, bright light of a rare snowy day in Albuquerque, the stark reality of our life hit me squarely in the face. The window I was looking out of oddly spanned from floor to ceiling, and there were no shades to draw down. Even though we were on the fifth floor, I could look down at the cars searching for a parking space in the lot below, and further out, view the traffic on the busy street.

I thought how each window on this side of the building contained a person with a specific life crisis going on at this same moment in time. Each one had a story of a battle raging on concerning their health. We were not the only ones, but now, I felt very alone. My husband was vulnerable. One of the few times of his entire life.

Around 11:15 a.m. the cart arrived to take Jim downstairs for the spinal. We had been told it was a painful procedure. With mixed feelings, I watched him being wheeled away. This test could hold the answer. *How much more could he endure?* The headache still persisted with a vengeance.

In the time he was gone, I called my boys and let them in on the news. Strangely, I hadn't called them before now. One day had led into another, and without a conclusion to give them, I kept putting it off. They each lived more than twelve hours away, and all three had jobs and other family responsibilities. I didn't want to cause them stress until we knew what we were dealing with. Although I still had no answers, I suddenly needed to hear their voices. I needed their support.

About two hours later, my husband returned. He was freezing cold, after being left out in the hall on a gurney for at least forty-five minutes of that time. The test was over, but there was no one to wheel him back. My protective instincts kicked in, and within minutes, another warm blanket arrived to wrap around his shaking frame.

Suddenly, Jim began to laugh and shake his head. He was finally losing it. But as I listened to his story, I began laughing too—a brief moment of relief. He related how he was being wheeled down the hallway, up the elevator, and into our unit. As he passed the room next to ours, he glanced over into the room and, to his utter surprise, there was his wife sitting in the bed with her top off.

Just as he was getting over the shock, he was wheeled into his room to see his wife, fully clothed and anxiously waiting. This was the beginning of the morphine hallucinations which continued for at least two full weeks after we got released. Almost as an aside, Jim said his pain was subsiding.

I stopped and looked at him closely. "You mean your headache is going away?"

"Yes, it is . . . ." he said, with wonder in his voice.

I went out to the hall and across to the nurses' station. We knew each other quite well by this time. After informing her that Jim was telling me his headache was fading, she began to shake her head knowingly. "I have seen this happen before after a spinal tap. The fluid is drawn from the spine, the pressure is released from the brain, and the pain is gone."

Wow! I walked quietly back to our room to find my husband peacefully sleeping, and I immediately saw the stress released from his body. His face was relaxed, his body was still, and I began to feel a huge relief wash over me. Prayers were being answered. Now to hear the results of the test.

When the doctor made his rounds that evening, I could sense there was good news. He confidently walked into the room with a smile and relayed the news that everything looked good. By this time, Jim had experienced several pain-free hours. It was a sudden turn-around and seemed to be lasting. As thankful as I was, I still had one main question: *what caused all the pain in the first place?* A mystery of medicine. No definitive answers. But we were being released with instructions to come back if the headache returned. In addition, we needed to keep the sleep clinic appointment in a couple of weeks.

We drove home at almost midnight. I never knew people were ever released late at night. Welcome to the world of insurance limitations. The worst part of the whole ordeal occurred when the nurse came in to remove the tape around the IV. Jim yelped and carried on like a wounded animal. At one point he jerked his arm out of the nurse's grasp and strongly reprimanded her not to rip his skin off!

If only someone would invent painless tape that holds an IV in securely. Anyone with hairy arms must have had the same painful trauma—not a good exit experience, but finally the ordeal was over and we were headed home. The soft familiar bed we fell into an hour and a half later felt like heaven!

Chapter 5
The Little Morphine Men

"BARB, DO YOU SEE THAT LITTLE MAN sitting in the corner?"

We were in for an interesting, entertaining, and at times chilling two weeks. The morphine people came out of the woodwork when least expected. Jim would catch a movement out of the corner of his left eye. It was a series of flashes of bright lights. He handled it so much better than I did. He knew it wasn't real and began to use his always-ready sense of humor to dispel the crazy images. They would pop up out of the ditches as he drove the quarter mile over to the shop. Needless to say, he didn't drive any further than that. As long as he kept it in perspective, he was safe. I probably would have swerved into the ditch to hit the suckers! Every evening he would relate the new and creative ways they would appear.

At home, as we relaxed in our recliners, I began to feel like I was in a horror movie. My husband began to frequently see the flashing red lights he described as "exactly like the rotating flashing light atop a police car."

I had called the neuro doctor the second day, and the explanation seemed feasible. The small bleed found on the MRI could have affected the vision in the left eye temporarily. We scheduled a visit to an optometrist. The rest of the hallucinations were sometimes experienced by people who had taken in a large quantity of morphine. That certainly applied!

The single most radical, disquieting occurrence happened one night as we settled into bed. After our nightly prayers together, (which had lengthened considerably as I fervently asked God to take the weird men away), we were drifting off to sleep. All at once, Jim came up out of bed like a shot!

"What's wrong?" I shrieked.

Jim began to laugh uncontrollably. One of those little guys came up over the end of the bed, bringing the cover with him. After getting right in front of his face, the guy had peeked over the blanket, then suddenly disappeared!

I was shaken, Jim was highly amused. Par for the course. At least he was handling this with reason. On the other hand, I began to wonder about the edge of sanity. Not his, but mine.

Gradually the hallucinations diminished. and life began to return to a sense of normalcy. Best of all, the headache never returned. We both began to breathe easier. The day had arrived for the sleep clinic appointment. It seemed like almost an afterthought now, and probably unnecessary.

Nevertheless, we kept the appointment, and Jim was off again to another interesting night of tests. I drove him over to the clinic around 7:00 pm. He was to take his pajamas, a book or his choice of soothing music, and anything else that relaxed him. As I drove up to the door, he jokingly told me he needed his cuddle bunny to stay. With a smile, I gave him a quick kiss and told him to sleep well, and I would return at 6:00 a.m.

Over an hour into Albuquerque, the drive back home in the dark, a short night, and back to the city the next morning. I began to recall why I had decided to work on the farm rather than commuting around a hundred and forty miles per day in order to find a good job. I had left the nine-to-five world behind after moving to New Mexico. It was a new life. With all three boys grown and independent, Jim and I had entered the empty nest portion of our marriage in an interesting position. Not only were we spending evenings alone together, we were also working side by side on the farm every day. Actually, it fit perfectly.

My early days were rooted in farming, being raised on a family farm. I loved the communion of peace and solitude I found day after day in my swather cab. During the past ten years, I had experienced the privilege of encountering golden eagles, wild newborn antelope, coyotes sprinting across the field, along with rabbits, skunk, and deer. I loved eating lunch with my husband in the pickup cab in the middle of the hot summer days, and the satisfying feeling of pulling our work boots off together in the glider outside our front door after a long fulfilling day of honest work. I would later cherish those days together more than I ever thought possible.

Back in Kansas, where we had lived for over fifteen years, we virtually saw each other only on nights and weekends, and much of the time, not many hours then. I worked full-time at a commodity brokerage business, and twenty-six miles away, Jim managed a large irrigated farm. He unequivocally was the hardest-working man I had ever known.

Raised with a work ethic by a father who oftentimes worked three jobs, Jim had picked up that quality to the bone. As a farmer, he had the opportunity to practice it to the ultimate. And live it he did! There was not another worker throughout all the years of his profession who could outlast Jim. I witnessed again and again Jim's dogged never-give-up determination. I saw it in the three days he would go without sleep when he was up baling the alfalfa at just the right moisture level while his hired men were grumbling because they had to work ten hours straight.

I saw it on many occasions when he would persistently keep working on a broken-down piece of equipment until he figured out a way to fix it, long after his workers had gone home to their families. I have seen it as he climbed back on a tractor in the early hours to rake the hay after a worker failed to show up for work, even after he had baled hay all night long. Or get on a loader to help unload the bales coming off the fields into the hay sheds so the new bales would not be exposed to the weather.

I witnessed his dogged determination when he would survey a field shredded by a hailstorm just when the tall leaves of corn were ripe for harvest, and when the hot New Mexico winds had turned the new shoots of corn plants into dry withering stubs.

I had watched him climb up on the tractor to plant the whole field over again. I saw it through droughts, tornadoes, hail, flooding, and fires. Through hard financial times and sick children. Through failure and disappointment. He never gave up. He always lived by the words I heard his Grandma D. speak many times: "Where there's a will, there's a way."

Jim was impatiently waiting for my arrival the next morning, and, as always, very anxious to get back to the farm. He had very interesting news to tell me. It had taken him several hours to get to sleep, even though his normal exhausted state helped. Jim was always a light sleeper and did not do well in strange surroundings.

He had not fallen into a normal pattern of sleep until about 11:00 p.m. About three hours later, the technician awakened him and told him he had all the input he needed, not realizing Jim was without a vehicle to drive himself home. Although he could not discuss the details of his findings, he did tell him without a doubt, he was a classic sleep-apnea case.

We had an appointment with the sleep doctor a few days later. He told us in the three hours of graphic pattern testing, Jim's breathing had stopped a total of about seventy times! He explained how, in a patient with the condition, the muscle holding the throat open for absorbing oxygen relaxes and closes off the normal route of air entering the body. After a short period of time, a reflex action causes the patient to gasp and start breathing again. But during the span of non-breathing, blood pressure can shoot up suddenly, and the level of oxygen decrease. When this occurs many times over and over throughout the night, the purpose of sleep is abnormally interrupted, and the person will wake up more fatigued than when he went to sleep.

Who would have ever thought all the problems had been caused by a condition called sleep apnea?

Finally, an answer to some of the mysteries still rolling around in my head! Like the low oxygen level in the hospital. The bleed that could have been caused in the brain with a sudden rise of blood pressure. It began to fit together like a puzzle. And this doctor had a solution called a C-PAP machine. We could live with that if it took care of the problem.

This was easy for me to say, but in reality, Jim was the one who had to adjust to sleeping with a plastic, pressurized mask attached to a hose and a machine filled with water. He was the one who couldn't sleep on his stomach or toss and turn in the bed to get comfortable. He, the light sleeper, would have to adjust to the noise and the restriction and even the claustrophobic feeling of wearing a mask which eventually made his nose raw and required a constant adjustment. Months and months passed before he would say he honestly got adjusted to wearing it. But he never gave up, even when night after night he wanted to rip it off his head and just get comfortable. I praised God we had found the solution.

Life took on a normalcy again. Both the hay and the corn were harvested, and the crazy hours of summer and fall were transitioning to the slower rhythm of winter. It was the time of year that enabled us to revitalize, visit family, regroup, and plan for the new awakening of spring. Quiet evenings of reading and watching tv by the fireplace. Time for evening walks with our St. Bernard, Samson, and our black lab, Molly. A drive into the gorgeous valley of Albuquerque where the tall cottonwoods along the Rio Grande had turned to bright oranges and yellows, where the almost perfect year-round climate remains constant. A movie and dinner or an outdoor concert in the amphitheater out in the middle of nowhere where our favorite country stars sang in the cool night air. Peace began to fill our hearts, and we could relax and enjoy our simple lives once more.

On a trip home to Kansas at Thanksgiving, a family matter resulted in my staying for a few weeks while Jim returned to New Mexico alone. It was a mutual decision we made together, and all was well. Jim would return to Kansas at Christmas where we would celebrate with all our extended family and return home to New Mexico. Although it was a personal sacrifice of time and separation, we both agreed God was in it.

God was definitely in it. These words turned out to be the biggest understatement ever!

Chapter 6

The Revelation

Late November, 2009

BARB HAD BEEN GONE ALMOST an entire week. I didn't like to sleep alone. It just wasn't the same not being able to reach over and touch her warm soft skin. For years, we had slept like two spoons stacked together, taking up only a fraction of the queen bed we lay in. A perfect fit of warmth and security.

Recent years had gradually changed our sleep positions. Hormones and hot flashes had caused my wife to want her space. I also identified with interruptions of sleep. During the night, I would get up to go out to the fields a few times to check the hay fields for moisture; this encouraged me to sleep further away so I wouldn't wake her as I arose.

My old back injury, and the bursitis that had developed in my shoulder caused me to toss and turn to find a comfortable position;

then, of all annoying things, I had been diagnosed with sleep apnea and had been ordered to sleep with an air mask over my face all night. I had half a notion to throw the stupid, confining contraption in a corner while Barb was gone and get back a semblance of comfortable normalcy. But she would have had a fit if she knew that I slept one night without it.

She was constantly asking me if I was wearing it every night during our frequent phone calls to one another, and besides that, I knew it was for my own good to wear it. If only I could get used to the swishing sound from the machine, the sealed tightness of the mask around my nose and mouth, and the restriction of the attached hose. Maybe by the time I got my wife back, I would be adjusted to it. I fell into a deep sleep of exhaustion.

"Wake up."

As I teetered between sleep and a state of alertness, I wondered if I had actually heard the words. I sat up on the side of the bed and took off the mask. I reached over and turned off the noisy CPAP machine and began rubbing my eyes.

All became intensely quiet. The loud tick-tock of the pendulum clock hanging on the dining-room wall was the only noise breaking the silence. Yawning and stretching, I started to get up and go to the bathroom and get a drink of water.

"You have less than two years to live on this earth. During the time remaining, love your wife and your family more deeply and completely than you have ever loved them before."

I sat back down on the bed hard. No, not audible. I looked around the room, half expecting to see an angel. I knew it was from the Lord, and there was no doubt about the message. It came across my mind and heart as real and full of truth as anything that could have been spoken out loud. It was heavily stamped upon my heart and across my consciousness. *How long did I sit there, bowing my head and trying to absorb what had just happened?*

I was certainly wide awake now. The words kept repeating themselves again and again in my mind. *I was going to die within two years?* I was not even sixty years old. Although I had been through a health scare earlier, other than a little inconvenience, I was living life normally again.

I had been raised to put work first. I had been taught that my job as a husband and father was to provide and take care of my family. I knew, throughout the years, this mindset had taken a toll on my wife and three boys, but it was like a drive within me I felt I almost didn't have any control over.

I knew, left unchecked, it eventually would have broken my family apart. When a man works sometimes eighteen hours a day doing hard, physical labor, there just isn't enough left to be the husband and father he needs to be. Over the years of our married life, the main disagreements between Barb and I had centered around the fact she was raising the boys virtually alone, and I was missing out on many of the golden moments of their lives.

The change-point came when I found Christ. When I surrendered my life to Him completely, I began to learn what my role as a man consisted of in God's plan and purpose. A few key men came into my life and taught me what a real man is. It is not who can work the hardest and keep going. A godly group of men introduced me to Promise Keepers, a nationwide organization dedicated to helping men to achieve the goal of being all God desires them to become.

I went to several weekend events in Dallas, Denver, and even a rally that covered the Mall in front of the Washington Monument in Washington, D.C. I began to get a grasp on God's picture of a man's role in His perspective: the biblical definition where the man leads his family by a loving example with wisdom and truth as his guide.

I remember coming home from one conference where I had learned about *blessing* my wife. The first night I was home, when we were getting ready to go to bed, I knelt by the side of our bed and asked her to sit close to me. I told her I wanted to give her a blessing and put my hands on her head and prayed. I began to see silent tears sliding down her cheeks, creating wet splotches on her nightgown.

She remained perfectly still until I finished, then she broke down and cried. "That is the nicest thing you have ever done for me!"

I began to realize at that moment what being a true man was all about.

But although becoming a Christian had softened my rough edges, I continued to battle the inbred pull on my life toward work. I still remained in the one career I knew and loved. The only way I knew to approach it was with hard work and long hours. It begged my full attention, never letting up on its continual demands for my time and attention.

A farmer's work is never done. This lifestyle is modeled around complete devotion and absorption of your entire life. The hardest years were when my wife worked in town twenty-six miles away and the boys were involved in school activities and sports in the same town. I tried really hard to make most of their games and important school accomplishments, but Barb was having to handle most of the load.

We were also heavily involved with our church, and I taught 3rd and 4th grade boys Sunday school every Sunday morning. So, even on Sundays, I was rising at dawn and checking all the irrigation systems before getting back to the house, showering, and jumping in the van with the family for the drive to town.

As irrigation systems don't always run like clockwork, there were frequently problems I would encounter that would cause a delay in our departure. Those mornings would cause me to speed over the back roads into town to make it on time. Our small-town deputy sheriff had a habit of sitting on that route on Sunday mornings. After stopping me and giving me a warning to "slow down" after my hasty explanation of why I was speeding, he finally stopped parking on that highway at that time. I think he just didn't have the heart to give a man a ticket for trying to make it to church on time.

Years later, one of the boys I had taught Sunday school to was interviewed as a senior student by the local newspaper. In his own words, he wrote about the farmer who had sacrificed his precious time to drive all the way into town and teach a little Sunday school group of boys every Sunday, and what an impact it had made on his life! I was stunned and extremely rewarded by that little interview. The article became worn and creased in my billfold all the years afterwards I carried it with me.

So, rewards would come when I made the extra effort to serve and learn about the Lord. My wife and I attended a Master Life class with some of our close friends from church, including our pastor and his wife. It was more than a struggle for me, as I have always had a mental block when it came to memorization.

Each week we were supposed to memorize several Bible verses. My group of friends encouraged and helped me practice this skill until I was able to accomplish the process and pass the nine-week class. I wanted to hide God's Word in my heart and mind. I was able to learn to do that with little cards I took out to the field with me and practiced with as I drove the tractor.

Most of all, during this class I learned to identify what my spiritual gifts were. I distinctly remember the night we sat together and talked about the gifts we saw in each other, as displayed in our lives. Mine were mercy, giving, and serving others.

These gifts had gotten me in trouble with Barb at times. There had been more than one instance when I had loaned out money to my workers after they had told me about a need they had, without clearing it with my wife first. Not the best idea, but sometime in the process, I almost always was given the opportunity to tell them about the Lord and how they needed to get Him involved in their life. I would share with them how He had made all the difference in mine. In a very desperate situation when my marriage almost crumbled, I reached out and pleaded with God for help, and miraculously, He did!

I would tell them that through experience, I had found following Him was the best way to get through all the troubles of this life. It steers you around and away from some of those really bad situations. It gives you something to grab hold of instead of turning to drugs or alcohol for the answers. I believe it actually got through to some of those men. I saw their language cleanup and a new respect come over them. Some started taking their families to church.

After bailing one man out of jail, I was able to really reach him in his desperation. He had hit rock bottom and no one else would help. He was open and ready for a changed life. He had some skills and talents I could use on the farm. I was usually ready to give a guy one more chance. Sometimes they grabbed hold, and sometimes their past habits overtook them again.

Many years ago, when Barb and I were in Oklahoma leasing a dairy farm, one of those *last chancers* showed up out of nowhere asking for a job. He had been hitch-hiking aimlessly across the country after his life had completely fallen apart upon his return from the Vietnam War. Before the war, he was a skilled, licensed plumber in a big city with a wife and two children. Now, he was a ravaged alcoholic with only dim memories of what it meant to live a meaningful life. Rage had filled up the empty places of his life, and the scars on his body were there to prove it.

When I brought him in the door one night to feed him a hot supper and send him on down the road, I could see the frightened look on my wife's face as this stringy-haired, dirty, thin shell of a man followed me into the kitchen.

"Do we have enough extra to share some supper tonight?"

There was a moment of hesitation before Barb reached up in the cabinet for another plate. By this time, she knew me too well. It wasn't the first time I had showed up unexpectedly with a stranger. And she had a way of drawing someone out and getting them to talk about themselves. Her perception about a person was seldom wrong, and I learned to trust it.

The next two hours went by quickly as Steve told us his life story. Much later we came to realize that, except for the grace of God, any of us could be where Steve found himself. A few wrong choices mixed in with some tragic circumstances can bring anyone to desperation.

Steve was highly intelligent and came from a wealthy family. As we later experienced, he was highly skilled and extremely loyal. He ended up working for us for several months, and we took him to church with us every Sunday. We knew he often teetered on the edge. He told us about the flashbacks of indescribable horror that came back to haunt him in the night. He talked to me privately about being a tunnel rat in Vietnam, and shared horrific, unspeakable stories of what he had lived through. He told us how the war had ripped his family away from him, and how alcohol had taken the rest of his life, including his job. We became good friends, and I hoped the Lord would inhabit and clean out the putrid areas of his life.

One Sunday morning, he didn't show up for church. That afternoon, I went to town to search for Steve at the house he was living in. After not getting an answer, I stopped by another worker's house to see if he'd seen him. He had been with him at the local bar the night before, and evidently, all hell had broken loose. Someone had provoked Steve into a fight, the rage had appeared, and Steve had severely beaten a man. Steve had run out before the cops got there, and it was the last he had been seen. It turned out to be the last time we ever saw Steve, too.

Several years later, an official letter appeared in our mailbox from a judge asking me to tell him what I knew about Steve. Steve had given my name as a character reference. I not only wrote a letter for him, but also called the judge and talked to him personally about Steve. I asked the judge if maybe he could be the one to help Steve get one last chance, of course, after needed rehab and justice for whatever trouble he was in. I never knew the end of Steve's story, but I sure hope it turned out well for him. He was a person of value, a man with great potential, and I know God loved him and wanted the best for him, too.

Ironically, although I extended mercy to others generously, I tended to be rather hard on my wife and children. I expected them to be tough and work as hard as I did. Two of my three boys got burnt out on farming by that approach. The third son was so much like me: he thrived in that environment. Although I became more tender with my wife as the years went by, I was still too hard on her and I knew it. She had followed me faithfully as the years went by and always allowed me to chase my dreams. I wanted desperately to own my own farm someday and tried a couple of times to fulfill that dream—each time without success.

The dreams took us from central Kansas to southern Oklahoma, back to western Kansas, and finally to central New Mexico. By the time the job of managing a huge farm in New Mexico came up, I had finally accepted the hard fact that owning my own farm was not going to happen. Financially, it was next to impossible unless you inherited the land. Farm expenses for equipment, fertilizer, and irrigation had skyrocketed as the decades went by.

Along with the loss of my lifetime dream, another perspective had eased the pain. I could manage a farm the way I chose and wake up every morning to the way of life I loved. But instead of worrying principally about the finances, my main goals were to produce the best crops around; work day by day in the dirt; achieve the challenges and goals I set for myself and my employees; and earn a good salary. When I looked at it that way, I was in the best position.

Barb worked in a full-time job in town for about twenty years of our marriage, and although I supported her in this, she had gotten little actual help from me with the housework, cooking or child-raising. In two of the places we moved, she had worked right alongside me on the farm, driving tractors, taking care of baby calves, and whatever else I had asked her to do.

Although she knew without a doubt I loved her, my expectations of her were sometimes out of reason. I tended to treat her like I treated the other hired men instead of placing her in a position of honor. I had often neglected telling her how I truly appreciated her, but constantly bragged about her to my friends.

When we moved to New Mexico, she had willingly decided to work with me on the farm so we could spend more time together. It turned out she became the only person on the farm who I completely trusted to cut the alfalfa with the thirty-foot, triple-section swather attachment we had put on our big Claas harvester. She was proud of this accomplishment, and I was proud of her, as there are many different, complicated controls and functions you constantly need to be watching as you cut.

Barb came to love the outdoor experience with nature and often talked about the many animals she encountered in the fields. For the most part our lives were good, but the old habit of holding my personal emotions at arm's length still put a damper on our marriage and the intimacy we should have had.

Is this the reason the Lord had spoken to me? Is it possible I was being punished? Had I not shown my boys and Barb how much I cared for them enough? If I changed my actions and words, would God change his mind about taking me so soon?

All of these thoughts came through my mind in a tangled jumble that night. I had three more long weeks alone before I would go back to Kansas over Christmas to bring my wife back home. Three very long weeks during which I searched, I agonized, I doubted, and I prayed.

During the second week, I was scheduled to go over the border from El Paso to Juarez, Mexico to have some dental work done. A neighbor and good friend of mine told me about the dental clinic he had been going to for years there, and he had talked me into going with him one time. It was surprising to find this was a thriving business in which hundreds of Americans participated in regularly. Not only was the dental work cheaper, but it was done quickly and efficiently in a modern, sterile clinic just across the border.

However, since the last time I was there, conditions in Juarez had changed drastically. Recently, many shootings and kidnappings had been reported, and the drug cartel was running rampant. It was probably why I waited until the last possible moment before the dental van came to pick me up in El Paso to call and tell Barb I was going across. With good reason, as she had a fit over the phone when I made that last-minute call—especially when she found out I was doing this alone without my friend's accompaniment.

Why had I decided to keep the appointment? Especially after I couldn't get any of my friends to ride along with me. Maybe I was feeling reckless. I had wanted to go to a big city to buy something special for Barb for our upcoming anniversary, but I could have shopped in Albuquerque. Maybe I just needed to be away from the farm for a couple of days to have more time to think about what had happened to me.

After talking to my wife, I began to question my sound judgement, but it was too late. The van was almost at the motel, and I had driven all this way already. Was I tempting God? Was I shaking my fist at Him and telling Him to go ahead and prove Himself? If I was close to being taken out of here, was I somehow telling Him to go ahead and do it quickly? Suddenly I was afraid He might just follow through. I humbly bowed my head and asked for His protection.

I had gotten the idea of buying Barb a new wedding ring. Although we had celebrated our big anniversaries over the years by going on some special trips, I knew she had longed to have the cheap golden bands, the only ones we could afford to buy each other as teenagers, replaced by a real diamond. She always told me it didn't matter, but I hoped this surprise would show her how much I really cared about her.

I found just the right one with three diamonds representing the past, present, and future, as well as the three sons God blessed us with. I sure hoped she would love it. I even came up with a fun idea of how to surprise her with it on our anniversary in February. Just the thought of seeing her face when she opened it caused me to smile. Maybe it was also one way of being obedient to God. It felt good and right. We were planning a special cruise to celebrate our 40th anniversary. I would give it to her on that day out at sea. It made me smile again to think about her reaction.

Chapter 7
The Kodak Moment

THE WEEKS BETWEEN THANKSGIVING and Christmas went by quickly. I had done the right thing by helping my family out in their time of need. Before I knew it, Christmas arrived, and I was ready to get back home to my life in New Mexico. We drove the two-and-a-half hours up to our oldest son's for Christmas Eve and Christmas day before making the long drive back to New Mexico.

Unexpectedly, Christmas Eve found us alone for a few hours. Our son was going through a long and emotional divorce, and his estranged wife and he were feeling their way through the first holidays. They had decided to spend a couple of hours together with their children to make the time as normal as possible for the kids' sake.

The fireplace was roaring, the Christmas tree lights were glowing, and Jim and I were feeling the joy of reuniting after a month apart.

There was something extraordinarily special about the evening. After the hustle and bustle of the day's activities, quiet permeated all around us. For a while, we just sat and enjoyed the crackling of the fireplace.

Jim broke the silence, "Shall we go ahead and exchange our presents to each other?"

It suddenly hit me that this would be a perfect stolen moment before the Christmas chaos returned. "I was about to suggest the same thing. Besides, I can't wait to see this present you hinted to me about over the phone. Remember when you said you bet it would be better than what I got you? Well, I have been curious about it for the past few weeks."

We went and retrieved our separate packages.

"You go first!" I proudly exclaimed.

I couldn't wait to see the look on his face when he opened his present. I had found a portable DVD player Jim could watch his movies on when we went on trips or as he was lying in bed. We only had one television in the house in the living room, and I knew he would just love this idea. He smiled and looked up at me with a special glint in his eye after he had opened the present.

"That was really great, Barb. But we'll see if you still think yours was the better present."

He reached down and handed me an average-sized box. As I stared at the opened box, I tried not to appear disappointed. In fact, I mustered up a real excitement about the traveling steam iron, expounding on how much I could use it to touch up wrinkled clothes from being smashed down in suitcases on airplane trips. He described in great detail how a guy was demonstrating them in the mall in El Paso, and how much he thought I would love it when he ran across it--how he knew he had found just the perfect gift for me for Christmas. I continued to smile and look at the little iron as if it was the most precious gift I had ever received. He seemed to be so proud of himself for the discovery of such a unique, clever find.

"You were right, Honey. Your gift is much better than mine," I said with complete sincerity in my voice.

"Oh, and did you look in the bottom of the box at the special filler that came with it?"

I got prepared to do more bragging on the ingenious one-of-a-kind item. As I reached down to retrieve the funnel, I saw another little box in the bottom corner. As I pulled it out, a huge grin spread across Jim's face.

"What is this?"

Waves of realization began to spread across my brain as I looked at the little velvet jewelry box I was holding.

"Well, open it, and see!"

By this time, he was beginning to chuckle. You could have truly knocked me over with a feather when I slowly opened the hinged box and saw the most gorgeous gold ring with three shining diamonds sparkling out into the room. I slowly took the ring over to him and suddenly burst into tears! I had proudly worn the simple 10-karat gold band with the tiny starburst pattern circled around it for almost forty years.

Then one fateful night, I had taken it off and laid it on the edge of the microwave table in the kitchen of our house in Kansas as I was scrubbing some rusty pans with scouring powder. Later, as I walked by that little cart, I bumped it. The ring fell off, and my curious kitten, that happened to be standing right there, saw it hit the floor and roll. With one swat of his paw, he knocked the ring down into the floor vent. My kitten stood over it and peered down into the vent to see where his new toy had suddenly gone. I ran and got a screw driver, removed the vent cover, and reached down as far as possible to retrieve the ring.

After shining a flashlight down into the vent, I realized the duct made a downward curve and the ring was beyond sight and reach. As my husband had already moved to New Mexico and I was by myself in Kansas for a few months, I had neither the means or the ability to be able to get it out. To this day, that ring is laying somewhere in an air duct in a little frame house in Kansas.

"Now do you still truly believe your gift was better?" Jim mocked with a sarcastic, teasing tone.

I slipped the ring on my finger and watched it sparkle brightly in the firelight. "It is perfect! Just beautiful! I couldn't have picked out anything I liked more!"

Tears coursed uncontrollably down my cheeks. He explained the symbolism of the three diamonds, and I cried harder. I wrapped my arms tightly around his neck and we held each other for a long time. In that moment, I felt closer to my husband than I had felt for years.

"I was planning on waiting until our anniversary trip in February to give it to you, but I just couldn't wait."

He truly seemed as excited as I was. It was a magical night. A magical couple of hours between a man and a woman who had been together for almost forty years of ups and downs and troubles and heartaches and joys and laughter. A couple of hours of getting back to the pure simple love between a husband and a wife. People refer to special times like these as "Kodak moments." A snap-shot of a rare, perfect moment in time you can find great joy in as you reflect on it.

Little did I know this memory would be one of those precious nuggets to look back on and cling to in the impossibly difficult times ahead of us. A special, glowing, happy time when all was well with the world.

Chapter 8
Badminton, Anyone?

January, 2010

AFTER CELEBRATING CHRISTMAS DAY with our family in Kansas, Jim and I drove back home. I was ready for a nice, quiet time of rest and recuperation—some real down time.

Thankfully, January was one of the slow months on the farm when my only responsibility was to do some record keeping and government reports. The rest of the time, I could relax and go back to my one personal fun indulgence. I had joined a group of other local people wanting to participate in regular exercise by playing indoor badminton three times a week. I unexpectedly found it to be about the most fun, enjoyable activity I had ever done.

It was a great mix of both local and newly-transplanted retirees, all with a positive attitude, and all there for the same reasons. The group had been formed by a man who had found the great fun and challenge of badminton through the organization of Senior Olympics. It had caught on and continued even after the man had moved.

I soon found there was a great deal of skill and strategy involved in the game to make it challenging and competitive. It fit perfectly with my personality, and I had progressed to a competitive level where we participated in tournaments across the state and beyond. I had even gone to the national level one year in California. This was my time of complete and unbridled fun and missing a month of it had been tough.

One day, the second week after I had been back home, I woke up with a strange feeling all over. I had a nagging sore throat and dull buzzing headache. But most of all, I felt this overwhelming sense of fatigue. Great! I didn't want to be sick now! I must be coming down with the dreaded flu bug, even though I had gotten a flu shot back in October. As is my usual style, I pushed the sick feeling to the back of my mind and continued to get ready for my fifteen-minute trip into town to play badminton for a couple of hours. But after about an hour of strenuous play, I was extremely fatigued.

It had taken me several months to finally build up my endurance time in this high New Mexico altitude of 6800 feet. I never thought my lungs and heart were ever going to adjust to playing all-out for two solid hours. But I had finally reached that level and had never felt better in my life! By now, I had put in several years and truly was getting to the top of my game. I went home that day with the sinking feeling something strange was wrong with me.

By the end of the week, I was sitting in the P.A.'s office telling her all of my persisting symptoms. I was not feeling worse, but certainly not better. She ran some blood work and put me on an antibiotic. The strep test had come back negative, and she thought I might just have an infection in my throat. I completed the round of meds, and two weeks later I went back for a follow-up visit. I was not feeling any better. I still had the headache, the sore throat, the extreme fatigue, and no fever. Following another round of a different antibiotic, back I came again, still reporting the same symptoms.

"It must be a virus that has invaded your body, and it might just have to run its course."

"I know this is a crazy thought, but could a fifty-something-year-old woman get Mono?"

This weird thought had entered my head sometime in the middle of one of those midnight hours when the imagination ran wild and played tricks on my numb, sleep-deprived brain.

She shrugged and gave a quick laugh.

"Very unlikely, but not impossible. Let me go look it up."

I appreciated her for not just discounting the very idea and sending me back home with more advice about just resting and waiting some more.

After lying on the hard, tissue-covered examining table for another fifteen minutes, she returned to find me dozing. I found myself doing that a lot these days—dropping off to get a few minutes restless sleep during all hours of the day. "You can get Mononucleosis at any age, although the most common age is in the teen years. The good news is there is a blood test that will definitely tell us whether you have it or not. Let's draw some more blood."

Several days later, the test results were in. I tested positive for the Mononucleosis virus.

I was scheduled for an appointment to go back in for a consultation. *How on earth had I contracted this virus? How long would I be down with it, and what could I do to get it out of my system quickly? I didn't have time for this nonsense!*

I had an exciting trip to take in February for our big anniversary, and we had already put down a large deposit. We were far into the planning stages, so hopefully there was a medicine I could take to quickly get me back to my normal healthy state. And I had badminton to play, for Pete's sake! I never missed practice in the winter months when I was not out working in the fields. This was putting a big cramp in my lifestyle, and I wanted it to just vamoose!

"There is no medicine to attack this virus. It runs its course differently in each person who contracts it. The normal time period is about three months without complications. It can attack different organs of the body and cause other problems, but hopefully it won't happen in your case. All you can do is get plenty of rest, drink lots of fluids, and listen to what your body tells you. No excessive exercise, and we will monitor you week by week until it is gone."

I was stunned, but a little voice had been telling me I had Mono. Dr. Susan had just said it out loud. The eternal optimist part of me took over. *I would bounce back quickly. I was very healthy and my body would shake this off in no time. I might have to cut back badminton time to an hour three times a week.* By mid-February, I would leave this virus in the dust and celebrate with my husband on our long-awaited cruise!

God had other plans. By the next week, when I went back in for my appointment, Mono was kicking my rear. My appetite was not only shrinking rapidly, but when I did eat, strange symptoms were occurring all throughout my digestive system. My stomach would begin to rumble, role, and growl incessantly and loudly a few minutes after I ate. I started feeling nauseous, and the list of foods I could tolerate was rapidly shrinking.

After pulling myself up out of bed each morning, I found a trip to the bathroom and out to the kitchen left me exhausted. I looked in the mirror at a very pale, sickly woman with dim, lifeless eyes, and wondered who she was and where she had come from. Then I would stumble back to bed and sleep for a couple of hours, only to wake up and repeat the same thing all over again. The day of my appointment came and with it a fear I might not be able to drive myself in. How could this have happened to me in such a short period of time?

Badminton, anyone? I let out a short bitter laugh. An hour three days a week? I could barely push the buttons on the phone to tell my teammates I couldn't come.

Dr. Susan had been doing her homework. On the examining table, she began to push and prod on my tummy. There was an unusual tenderness on one side, and I described the odd digestive gymnastics my body had been performing. "We need to watch this carefully. With Mono, rarely the spleen comes under attack. It can cause an enlargement, and worse-case scenario, it can burst. If this was to occur, it could be a life-threatening situation. It appears yours might be swollen."

It would explain how poorly I was feeling, but I didn't want to accept what she said next. "You can't indulge in any strenuous exercise, which could put you in danger of this occurring. Each week, we will measure the spleen and determine if it is enlarging. Just go home and rest!"

Rest was all I had been doing, and I was already tired of it. With badminton completely out of the question, I resigned myself to riding this out. Thus, began a new reality for me called: The Isolation of Living Out Mono. Time seemed to stand still, and I was trapped inside my house with very limited choices of activities, menus, or ambitions.

Other than my short recovery time after a hysterectomy about ten years prior, I was the picture of health, very rarely down for more than a day or two. *How would my husband respond to this? Would he believe I truly could not function, even with the smallest household chores?* The doctor had indicated if indeed the spleen was involved, my recovery time could be extended to several months.

Jim's response was phenomenally incredible! I saw a tender, compassionate side of my husband he had rarely ever shown to me. He fixed my eccentric meals, making sure I was never out of cottage cheese, apple sauce, bananas, apple juice, and hot tea. He made sure I was supplied with an endless variety of reading material, which was my only source of pleasure. I wasn't able to stand the noise of music or television.

Without the slightest suggestion, he was doing laundry, cooking and cleaning up after himself, keeping the bathrooms clean, and stopping in frequently during the day between his work responsibilities to sit and chat and check to see if I needed anything. And, most of all, he was doing it without a single trace of resentment or displeasure. He was doing it out of pure love.

The months droned on slowly. My spleen had gotten enlarged and I had an extended recovery time. Needless to say, our anniversary cruise had to be cancelled. Each week my husband drove me to the doctor's office to be measured and poked and questioned. This case of mine was creating quite a stir at the clinic, as it appeared to be quite a rarity.

One week, a substitute doctor came and examined me, and spent some extra time reviewing my file, which had grown quite thick by this time. "This is something I've only read about, but never seen. I'll be interested to see how your case comes out."

Well, I was so glad I was giving these doctors some new experiences, but oh, how I was ready to be done with this condition! Over the weeks, I continued to lose strength, and the cloud of fatigue seemed to hang over my head persistently. My goal now was to be well enough to run the swather to cut the first cutting of alfalfa in mid-May. My son had brought my two granddaughters to visit over Easter to "cheer Grammy up." Although they fulfilled that purpose, I was so exhausted I had to spend most of the time in bed while they were there.

Both Jim and Chad pitched in and cooked all the food for the weekend. I got to enjoy watching the girls play and have fun with their Easter candy and gifts. I read the Easter story to them from my bed and talked about the real meaning of Easter. We sat out on the porch in the glider for a little while with Samson, our St. Bernard, at our feet.

Would I ever get back to my normal healthy state of energy where I could play games and go for walks with the girls and Samson? I began to empathize with bedridden folks and those going through long illnesses, confined to their homes and their rooms. What a small world your life can become when you are unhealthy. I told the Lord if He would get me through this, I would never take my good health for granted again.

The stack of books I read seemed to measure the length of time I had dealt with this illness. The stack grew higher and higher as the days ticked by. Friends from badminton and Bible study called and checked on me periodically or drove out to bring us a meal and visit for a little while. I continued to marvel at the cheerful, caring spirit of my husband as he patiently saw me through the long duration. I thanked God for the good man He had given me and vowed to never take him for granted after my recovery.

Spring arrived, and as the earth began to awake from its winter sleep, I found myself slowly waking up from the long winter of darkness I, too, had experienced. I had begun taking short walks down the road in the warm afternoon sun, with Samson plodding along beside me with his lion-sized gait. He seemed to sense I could not go fast or tolerate his straying into the fields for a short run after a jackrabbit. He was content to obediently keep pace with his weak mama, and faithfully stopped to take a breather when I needed a short break.

When he could, Jim joined us, and we would stroll slowly down the pivot road watching the alfalfa come to life and start its season of quick growth. The walks and conversation were pleasant and healing, and I began to hope again of a return to my previous state of health. These long months were not without good lessons learned, (mostly about patience), much introspection, and taking stock of my life and purpose.

I was ready to start fully living my good life once more. I was anxious to get out in God's beautiful green fields of alfalfa and start working alongside my husband. I just wanted life to be stable and normal once again.

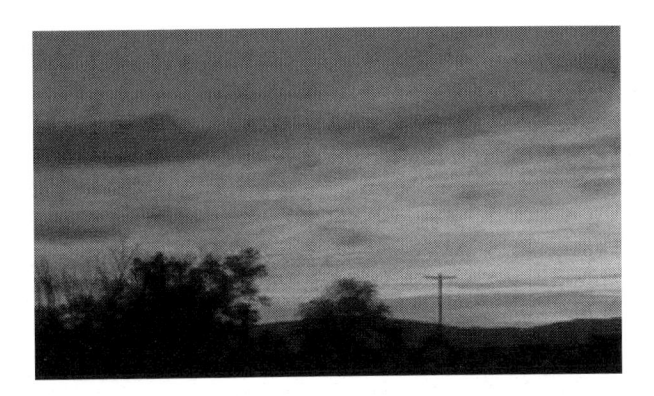

This June, sitting in the chair beside my husband's hospital bed, I thought about how ironic it had been that the place of 'normal' had only lasted a few short weeks. I finally regained enough stamina to cut the first cutting of alfalfa. Heavy fatigue followed a long day in the field, but it was a happy tired, a feeling of accomplishment and satisfaction. I would sit on the glider, unlace the work boots, stroke Samson's big head while he sat down heavily on my feet, and soak in the simple beauty of springtime on the farm.

The first cutting had gone well. The fields were tall, thick, and dark green. My machine had smoothly glided over the fields, eating up the plants and spitting them back out in thick, heavy, straight rows. The bright warm days of sunshine held out throughout the cutting, and not one field had gotten rained on. The rakes had gone over the rows, flipping the hay over to dry. It was condensed into fewer rows to be picked up by the balers, where it was transformed into packed, neat rectangles, and held together with knots of strong orange twine. The well-spent time of going meticulously over each piece of equipment in the winter repairing, greasing, and replacing wearing parts, had resulted in a smooth, hassle-free first cutting.

We were looking forward to our son coming in June for his normal 'farming fix.' His love of farming had stayed in his blood despite his different career choice because of the asthma and allergies that intensified when directly exposed to the grains and weeds on the farm. He had chosen to follow his other love, becoming an athletic trainer. It also required the great disciplines he learned from his father throughout his life while working alongside him from childhood through young adulthood. Like his dad, Chad had developed a strong work ethic, endurance, and dependability.

Having summers off with his job enabled him to come back and delve back into the hustle and bustle and craziness of the lifestyle he so enjoyed. He was Jim's right-hand man wherever he was needed.

Each year, Jim looked forward more and more to the time when his son could be there with him. It was so endearing to watch the two of them work side by side—dirty, sweaty, exhausted, and completely happy. This year, Jim had spoken several times about how much he looked forward to Chad's coming in June. It gave him such a boost.

Chapter 9
The Unfortunate Moment in Time

June 10, 2010

I TRIED NOT TO EVEN ALLOW my mind to go beyond the immediate problem at hand. This trip to the main downtown hospital with the neurology department where we had ended up the previous October was a no-brainer. We had gone through the learning process last time. I knew where to start this trip. I had called the neurologist and left a message stating Jim was having problems again, and we were bringing him in to be checked. Our personal P.A. had written out a referral to take with us to the hospital in case we needed it to get him admitted.

During check-in, the admitting person had asked us a question neither of us had ever encountered before. Did Jim have a Living Will? No, and we really didn't even know what it was. She patiently explained it was a booklet of pages dealing with detailed questions about what to do in case of a life-or-death situation that could occur during hospitalization, or in the case of an accident when you might be unconscious and unable to voice your wishes concerning your critical care. It was mainly about issues concerning life support and organ donation. We took the papers with us to fill out after being admitted.

As usual, the admittance process was fairly quick and easy. We had learned this happens whenever a head injury or condition are presented. Before long, we were once again on the fifth floor in the small Neurology Unit where we had been only seven months before. It was surreal being here again. We had gone through so much anxiety and uncertainty just seven months earlier, but it had seemed to conclude with a solution and what we thought would be the end of all the head issues.

The neurologist carefully had reread Jim's file and all that had taken place with the previous incident. We had filled him in on the sleep study results, and how the diagnosis of sleep apnea had resulted in successfully taking care of all apparent symptoms. We told him how the last few months were headache-free, and Jim's health had been good.

Then we got down to the specifics of the current episode. We explained in detail how the lapse in memory had taken place, followed by the gradual coming back to the senses, the light-headiness, and the headache that had suddenly become strong and persistent. We looked at him closely for an answer. *Why would this be happening? What could possibly be causing it?*

The doctor was also perplexed. "We will rerun some tests again. They should reveal what the real problem is. We will do another MRI. Hopefully we will have an answer shortly."

This time the morphine worked quickly to rid Jim of the terrible head pain. That was optimistic! Maybe this incident was just a weird fluke, and we could go home and forget all about it. Maybe Jim had just been working too hard and not getting enough sleep. The MRI was probably just a precaution and would not show anything out of the ordinary. We would spend the night, get the tests done in the morning, and be out of there by mid-afternoon.

This time there were two MRI's scheduled. One without contrast, the other one with contrast after injecting a dye into his brain. I was not really shook-up about the tests once Jim's headache was so quickly brought under control. We spent the evening watching TV with the sound down low, and afterward, I read my Bible by flashlight while Jim slept peacefully under the sleep mask we had brought with us to the hospital.

I had not called anyone except the workers back at the farm to let them know what we had found out about Jim. I folded out the sleep-chair and spread the blanket over me. Fatigue settled in over my body, and I went to sleep quickly with a prayer on my lips for good news tomorrow.

All the tests had been done without incident, and here we were, waiting to hear the results from the doctor himself. Why was it taking him so long? All hope of getting out of this joint tonight had vanished when he hadn't appeared by suppertime. We chalked it up to the possibility he had been called off to an emergency with another patient.

Thank goodness a basketball game was on to pass the time away. Periodically, I had stepped out of the room to check and see if there was any activity on the floor to indicate the doctor was making his rounds. The nurses had no answers to my frequent inquiries. They seemed as clueless as we were as to the doctor's whereabouts.

Hour after hour drug by, and I was about to give up on him making an appearance at all. Suddenly, around 9:25 p.m., he walked into the room without warning. By then, we were both so exhausted and frustrated, his entrance took us by surprise. His face was unreadable, but his words were soft and kind.

"I apologize for being so late in coming, but I do have the results of your tests. If you feel like making a little trip out to the nurses' station, I believe the easiest way to explain the results is for you to view them with me on the computer. Jim, do you feel like walking out there?"

"Yes, I'm really feeling so much better. The headache has been gone completely for most of the day. I'm just ready to get out of here for good!"

"Well, let's go look at these results, and then we'll talk about that."

It was eerie out there. The only lights on in the nurses' area were the blue lights of the computer screens. Where had the nurses disappeared to? It was as if we were the only people on the entire unit! There was total silence except for the gentle whirring of the computers. Following the doctor, Jim drug his IV unit along in his hospital gown and athletic shorts, and I trailed after the two feeling very strange and wary. The whole scene began to take on a suspicious air I could not begin to explain.

The doctor inserted a disk into one of the computers. "This is the picture of your brain from the back from the first MRI without contrast. Although there is a slight amount of swelling, it looks normal."

We both intently stared at the image. Ok, good. It looks normal.

He ejected the disk and stuck another one in.

"This is the same area of your brain done with contrast. Unfortunately, now something is showing up." There was an oblong area circled with a red marker over the image.

"One of the reasons we do the MRI with contrast is because a tumor won't show up on a standard MRI, but the dye will outline a tumor and become visible. When I first viewed this image, I saw the tumor just like you are seeing it now. I wanted to confer with another neurologist to make sure what I was seeing was correct. We also had a pathologist look over the images and confirm."

We remained frozen in place as we stared at the image. There was no bursting into tears. There was no shout of denial. There was only a need for more information.

"Unfortunately, this tumor is buried deep within the brain. That would mean we could not operate and remove it. It would be too dangerous and would do more damage than leaving it alone. After consulting with the pathologist, he agrees with us it has all the apparent characteristics of a malignant type of tumor called a glioblastoma.

"Unfortunately, it is a fast-growing tumor. Of course, the only way we can determine the exact type of tumor is by performing a biopsy. That can be dangerous, but it looks like it is feasible in your case. The brain surgeon will insert a very long needle down into the tumor and extract a sample big enough pathology can determine exactly what we are dealing with."

If I heard the word *unfortunately* one more time out of the doctor's lips, I would be physically sick. I had had enough of the word *unfortunately* to last a lifetime.

My logical, problem-solving side kicked in.

"Ok, if you are telling us this tumor is inoperable, how else can it be treated? Can it be shrunk down with radiation or killed with chemo?"

There was one more "unfortunately."

"Yes, I would recommend you immediately consult with an oncologist and radiologist. Unfortunately, IF this tumor is what we believe it to be, and we won't know until the biopsy is done, radiation and chemo can shrink the tumor for a period of time. But it will eventually begin to grow back rapidly. Let's schedule the biopsy as soon as possible. I do want to mention one more thing. When you were here several months ago, this tumor was not present. Do you have any more questions?"

Jim finally spoke. He had been completely silent up to this point. We had exchanged a couple of quick looks during the *unfortunatelys*, and our hands were tightly gripped to each other's. "Are you telling me I have brain cancer?"

I courageously fought back the first tears that instantly sprung to the surface of my eyes.

The doctor looked upon us with compassion. It almost set the tears bursting free, but somehow, I held them in.

"Let's take it one step at a time. I will get the biopsy scheduled and talk to you in the morning."

There was nothing left to say. I was glad the doctor had cleared the nurses from the station while he talked privately with us. I was glad he was open and factual. I was glad he had been truthful and direct and calm. It allowed me to be calm, too. I knew this had not been easy for him. This was not a good day in his life, as he knew the difficult journey we were about to embark on. We, at this point, had no idea.

We walked silently back to the room, and the silence remained as I went to the bathroom and prepared for another night in the hospital. Shock had overtaken both of us. Shock is God's way of insulating us when we cannot accept or deal with the situation at hand. It is kind and protective. It allows us to function in a cushioned sort of way. I could not even begin to accept this type of news in its totality. I walked over to Jim's bed and reached for his hand.

"Whatever lies ahead, God already knows about it. He will get us through it as He has always gotten us through. Just know I will do everything in my power to help you fight this."

"Was he telling us I have brain cancer?"

"Well, it sounds like that is what he was saying, but I'm not believing it until we get the tests back from the biopsy. We're going to have to take this one day, one minute at a time. God will help us through each step. It is the only sure thing I know right now."

I moved the chair/bed closer to his hospital bed and held onto his hand until my arm felt like it would fall off. At least Jim had sleep meds to mercifully knock him out. I was awake most of the night replaying every word, every detail of the surreal half hour when our lives were changed forever.

Each time I would drift off to sleep for a few minutes, I would suddenly jerk awake, only to question if I had dreamed the whole incident. Then each time, the reality would hit me like a brick wall— Yes, it was real, and I would again replay the scene over and over trying to make sense of it. I would then give myself a lecture of my own advice. 'One minute, one day at a time. Don't worry about tomorrow, for today has all the troubles we can deal with. Trust God. He cares about every tiny detail of our lives.' *Did I really believe those things? Yes, without a single doubt. Then give it all over to Him!*

"God, you know all about this mess. You know what we're feeling, what we're up against. You know how this is all going to shake out. I know you love us beyond comprehension, and you bring good out of all things. I trust you to lead us, guide us, direct us, and protect us. Give us courage and peace beyond understanding. Amen."

In that moment, peace beyond human understanding descended upon me. Tears began to flow, but they were tears of release. Releasing every single part of this whole huge burden over to a God who has the biggest shoulders in the world.

When daylight finally arrived, along with it came a stark, cold reality. This was huge. It wasn't just a small bump in the road that would temporarily cause inconvenience in our lives. This would change everything about us. From this day forward, we would be walking in a strange, uncharted, new world. I could already feel it as we waited to see what happened next. I could sense it in the way we were treated by the nurses as they moved in and out of the room performing their normal routine duties. The new information was either in the charts or the doctor had talked with them.

Most of all, I could feel the difference in the uneasiness that had settled in between my husband and myself. What was I supposed to say to him? What could I possibly say to make him feel better? There was a hurt look in his eyes that hadn't been there yesterday. I kept thinking all of our days and years of believing God's truths had led up to this day when we didn't just talk about what we believed. We had crossed a line where we had to live it out or abandon it. If we chose to live it out, we were going to have to trust Him unconditionally to care for us in every way, because we were completely helpless to change what had appeared on that MRI.

The doctor came in around 9:00 a.m. He had transitioned back into the role of professional neurologist. The vulnerability from the evening before had vanished, and he dealt factually with the process at hand:

"I have visited with the surgeon who will be performing the biopsy, and he has rearranged his schedule to get you in as soon as possible. He can operate on Monday morning. The sample will be sent to pathology, and as soon as they look it over, we will discuss the findings and set up a treatment plan. There is no reason to keep you here between now and Monday since your symptoms are under control, so I will sign the release forms, and we can get you out of here. Take it easy over the weekend and let me know if any problems come up. The nurse will give you pre-op instructions before you leave."

With that, he was gone. We were completely surprised we would get to go home before the biopsy was performed, but it was welcome news. Again, Jim had to endure the painful process of removing the tape around his arm from the IV. I collected our things quickly and helped Jim get dressed. He was wiped out from the whole ordeal of the last few days, both physically and mentally.

On the way home we discussed whether to call the boys and let them know what was going on, or waiting until after the biopsy to see for sure what we were dealing with. Jim thought it might be best to wait, but I told him they would want to know. If any of them could come, I would appreciate the support on Monday during the long waiting period.

After more discussion, we decided to call them. I dreaded making those calls. I could sense the circle of 'lives changed forever' expanding quickly, and I wanted to protect those whom I loved from feeling the pain as long as possible. We agreed to keep it confined to our children at this point until we had solid facts.

Usually, I love the feeling of walking back into my own home and looking forward to the sweet comfort of our own bed. But on that Thursday afternoon in June when the sun was brightly shining and the fields were tall and green with promise, all was askew with our world. It was hard to find comfort anywhere. A huge cloud loomed over us and we realized four days could be an eternity. Four extremely long days when the body and mind hung in suspense with complete uncertainty—when the gamut of possibilities swung from one extreme to the other.

Would we be one of the recipients of a direct miracle where the doctors would come out of the operating room with complete puzzlement because there was no tumor to be found? I didn't discount the possibility. I knew those kind of miracles still happen in this present day. Would the biopsy show the doctors were completely wrong, and what they had seen was a benign tumor that would prove harmless to Jim's brain in the future? Or would we find our worst fears realized? Would the biopsy prove Jim's tumor was malignant? As the pendulum of possibilities swung back and forth, my emotions did as well. Tears would alternate with hours of calmness, followed by tenseness that would overtake me, and finally complete and utter fatigue.

I distinctly remember the overwhelming drive to learn everything I could about brain tumors and the completely foreign word *glioblastoma* the doctor had used. I spent hours and hours on the computer looking at medical Web sites and reading every bit of information I could find concerning brain cancer. Depending on the type of glioblastoma tumor, treatment and prognosis could vary. The doctor had told us Jim's tumor looked to be a 'primary' type, one that had started and was contained to the brain, not metastasized or spread from another part of the body. Most of it was beyond frightening.

I read and reread information from many sites. It was almost more than I could comprehend. Brain cancer is rare. In fact, it is one of the rarest forms of cancer. How could my husband have gotten it? The only person close to me who had ever dealt with it was a first cousin who had died from it when she was a young adult, leaving behind two small children and a husband to raise them. But she had lived a state away and was many years older than me, so I was not directly affected. I just remember my mom telling me about how sad it was.

My brain ached with fatigue and stress. But I knew I had to make those difficult phone calls to our children. If any of them were going to come for the biopsy, I needed to give them time to make travel arrangements.

"Chris, this is your mom. I have some news to tell you about your dad. He's been in the hospital the last few days, and on Monday he will be having a biopsy to analyze a tumor the neurologist has found on an MRI that was performed. I hadn't called you before now because there wasn't any real news to tell. It all started when your dad came into the house the other night and told me he had a blackout of confusion about where to find an alfalfa field. He then got a headache that wouldn't go away, so I took him over to the hospital where he had gone last fall. I didn't know if you would be able to get away from work to come on Monday or not. It is entirely up to you, but I wanted you to know what's going on."

There was a time of silence before he spoke. "The doctor thinks it is a tumor? In his brain? Does he think it is serious? I am pretty swamped here at work, but if you need me to come, I will, Mom."

"Well, I am calling all you boys to let you know. Take some time to think about it, and then, get back to me. I know this is a shock to you just as it has been to your dad and me."

We talked some more about the string of events that had happened in the last few days, and then hung up.

This conversation was repeated two more times with the other two boys. I knew they all wanted to be there with me. I also knew each one had important job responsibilities and family obligations to consider. New Mexico was a long way from them all. It was the one down-side to taking this job. At times like this, how I wished we were closer to our children.

Chapter 10
The Moment of Truth

June 14, 2010

AS IT TURNED OUT, our son Chad was the one who was able to come and be with me through the biopsy. He arrived on Sunday, and we were up very early on Monday morning to drive into Albuquerque to the hospital. It was such a great feeling to have him with us. Just having him drive the SUV into the heart of the city was a huge relief. I knew I could have done it again with God's help but having Chad drive took a load of stress off my shoulders. A couple of my closest friends were going to be at the hospital along with two others to sit through the long waiting period.

During the prep time, after the anesthesiologist had come in and explained what would be happening, the main nurse assigned to our case asked Jim if he would like her to have prayer with him before he went in to surgery. Tears sprang to my eyes, and we both heartily accepted her offer. The prayer was beautiful and heartfelt, and we both needed it desperately. Trying to be brave, Jim had been joking and keeping things light. When the bed was wheeled in to pick him up for the trip down the hall into the operating room, I put on my bravest face. I smiled and told him we'd be waiting and would see him soon. I knelt to give him a kiss and told him I loved him, and he was whisked away.

I walked back down the hall and out to the waiting room to find Chad with a very heavy heart. I had a bad feeling the news would not be good. I knew whatever the outcome, we would find a way to deal with it. I am a fighter and I would do everything in my power to meet this challenge head on. I also knew without a doubt God had this. He already knew the outcome, and if it turned out to be bad, He would get us through it. But knowing this fact wouldn't keep me from praying every minute during the next long hours that the tumor just wouldn't be there.

We had been told it could take up to three hours for the biopsy, as the tumor was deep within the brain, and it would be a very tedious procedure. The doctor would come out and talk to us as soon as he successfully got a sample of the tissue and let us know how it went. We spent the time visiting about various topics and, as people are inclined to do, my friends and the other couple shared several personal stories. My mind would be distracted for a few minutes listening to their conversations, then I would jerk back to the seriousness and reality of what was happening.

My husband was down the hall in an operating room having a brain surgeon plunge a very long needle into the depths of his brain, drawing out the small sample of tissue that would determine our future and Jim's very life! Chad was painfully quiet and withdrawn.

One man was right in the middle of telling a rather humorous account of a personal incident when I looked up to see a tall doctor standing beside us. He still had the green paper cap covering his hair, and his face mask was tucked into his white coat pocket. I tried to focus my attention completely on his words.

"Your husband is doing fine. We just completed the biopsy and the tissue sample is being sent to pathology now. We will also send a sample on to another lab to confirm the results. The tumor seems to conform in every way to the initial analysis we made from the MRI. I can almost certainly tell you it looks like a *glioblastoma multiformme tumor*. The pathologist will be able to tell you exactly the stage and type."

"Could you tell if it is a malignant tumor?" I wanted to know the whole truth.

"If it is a glio multiformme in the place it is located deep within the brain tissue, it will almost certainly be malignant and fast-growing. But let's not put the cart before the horse. The lab reports will be conclusive, and you should have those results in the next couple of days. I'll have them come out and get you when Jim gets into recovery."

He turned and walked briskly away. Short and direct. I didn't detect the same compassion I had experienced with the neurologist, but I did appreciate the honesty.

What happened next was shocking. Without missing a beat, the man sitting next to our dear friends picked up his story right where he had left off, as if the news that had just devastated our lives had not even happened. As he arrived at the punch line of his story, I felt another punch in the gut.

Suddenly, my son jumped up out of his chair and rushed out of the waiting room into the hallway. I immediately ran out after him, finding him broken down in sobs. I grabbed hold of him and we both wept together, clinging to each other for a while. My friend had followed and stood with us, placing her loving arm on my shoulder. Her touch was filled with compassion. At the time, all I could think about was trying to grasp what the doctor had just laid on us, and how I could somehow comfort my hurting child. In the months to come, I would reflect on the absurdity of the incident. How unexpected and bizarre it was that the ones whom I expected to give the most support and comfort were the very ones who seemed least compassionate.

I felt betrayed and hurt and insignificant. It took me a long time to forgive the insensibility, but somehow, I have. In the long run it taught me just how important it is to be present and sensitive to the needs of others who are suffering through a tragedy. It taught me to truly empathize and share that person's heartache in the moment.

As Jim awoke in the recovery room, I struggled with what I should tell him. Even though the surgeon seemed pretty sure of the result, there was the outside chance he could be wrong. Funny how desperately we cling to those small glimmers of hope whenever possible. Human nature is strong. The will to live is powerful. And optimism persists until proven otherwise. I would wait until the tests were completed and we had gone to see the neurologist, who would explain the results in detail.

Right now, I just wanted to take Jim home and let him recover for a few days from all the trauma of the past few. I needed to regroup and pull myself together also, especially considering what could loom before us.

Besides the understandable fatigue from all he had been through the past few days, Jim seemed to be okay. He wasn't experiencing any more episodes of forgetfulness or confusion. In fact, it was almost impossible to keep him from resuming his job at full throttle.

Perhaps the most difficult task at hand was to go and have an honest talk with our bosses, the owners of the farm we managed. They had a right to know exactly what was going on. Although we had no idea where all this was going, they needed to be completely informed concerning what might be ahead. They were both shocked and sympathetic, just asking us to let them know as soon as possible about the pathology report.

With each person we talked to, it began to become just a little more real for us both. Personally, I drifted alternately in and out of shock, denial, and stark reality those couple of days. Jim kept his thoughts mostly to himself, turning to the refuge of absorbing himself relentlessly in the activity of the farm. I'm sure not one full minute of the next few days went by without our thoughts returning again and again to the results of the biopsy. I truly began to pray without ceasing, pleading with God to somehow turn this situation around for us.

On Wednesday morning, we got the phone call. We were contacted by a different neurologist's office and scheduled for a consultation on Thursday afternoon to go over the results. By then, the second lab from another state would also have sent their own set of results to the new doctor.

The next day, sitting across the desk from the doctor, I reached for Jim's hand as we both stared at the papers spread out before him. This was the moment of truth, and I braced myself. I physically felt every muscle in my body tense up as he cleared his throat to speak.

"What we are dealing with is a brain tumor with a long medical name. Officially, it is called a Type IV Glioblastoma Multiformme. It measures a little over four centimeters and is oblong in shape."

He pushed the papers toward us so we could see a physical diagram of the brain with the tumor drawn in. "It is located deep within the right side of the brain in the area that controls eyesight, balance, and logic perception. Right now, it is perhaps pushing up against those areas, but has not begun to cause major problems. What we need to do is to reduce the size of the tumor as much as possible through a combination of radiation therapy and chemotherapy. Our advice would be to set up these treatment goals as soon as possible beginning with appointments with both a radiologist and an oncologist, which we can set up for you as early as next week."

I don't believe I had swallowed, blinked, or moved a muscle since his mouth had opened to speak. I remember intently looking into his eyes and concentrating with all my being on his every word.

"Is the tumor malignant? Is this cancer we are talking about?"

It came out bluntly, but at this point, what was the use in trying to mince words? We were here to find out what we were dealing with.

"Yes, this is a malignant type of tumor. It is also fast-growing, which is why we need to get started on treatment right away."

"We both like to understand as much as possible about the situation as we can. So, with the treatment and the reduction of the tumor, will it then begin to grow back? Can you knock it completely out with the radiation?"

My husband, always a person of few words, was trusting me to ask all the questions. I knew he wanted to know the whole truth as I did. We were both realists when it came right down to it.

The doctor seemed a little reluctant to be completely forthright. I'm not sure he was prepared to deal bluntly with all the facts at this point. Perhaps he felt it was better to deal with the reality a little at a time. Too bad. He was going to be put on the spot. "The radiologist can give you better statistics than I can about the percentage of reduction you can expect. But to answer your question, no, the tumor will not be completely reduced, and will begin to grow again at some point."

"Okay then, let's get down to the brass tacks of the situation. Approximately how long does my husband have to live? I realize you can't be specific, but you must have a pretty good estimate? We need to know what kind of time we are talking about here."

I am pretty sure not too many people ask that question on the initial visit. But the doctor seemed to realize, finally, we really did want to know the facts.

"It can vary, but the average time seems to fall between eighteen months to two years, with very few making it as long as three to four years."

I swallowed hard, but the next question came out quickly. "Since we have no knowledge about this type of cancer, can you explain to us how it concludes? What happens at the end?"

At last, he seemed satisfied we really could take the honesty, and without hesitation, he relaxed a little. "Surprisingly, the end is easier with brain cancer than with many other types of diseases. There is not the painful trauma such as occurs with a major heart attack. The brain cancer patient begins to sleep more and more toward the end, and finally just drifts off into a coma."

As difficult as it had been to ask, I was glad I had. It gave us both just a little bit of peace in this horrible, life-changing, few minutes of catastrophic bad news.

Chapter 11
The Referral

Several Days Later

THE APPOINTMENTS WERE SET UP and we were bracing ourselves for the long ordeal. We would have to make many, many trips back and forth to Albuquerque for a number of weeks during the first round of treatments. We first met with the radiologist, who told us exactly what he would be doing to reduce the size of the tumor. He gave us the estimate of how many treatments it usually takes for the first round of radiation, explaining the amount a person can safely endure had been tested thoroughly.

The next appointment was set for the end of the week with the oncologist, who would explain all the ins and outs of the chemotherapy. In between the two appointments, I returned to the relentless pursuit of knowledge from the computer. It seemed like I was driven to discover a miracle in the middle of this horrible tragedy we were living in.

In the process of looking up information on treatment, I came across a site that peaked my interest. It talked about a group of facilities opening up across the United States using a type of radiation treatment that was more precise in targeting the cancer cells.

Only a few of these facilities had opened, but one was located only a couple of states away from us in Oklahoma. The draw was that this treatment more precisely hit the cancer cells without spreading out the radiation to normal cells. Less healthy cells were damaged or killed. This was particularly appealing when it came to brain cancer; not endangering the damage of brain functions close by the tumor area. The more I read, the more I was drawn to the explanation and logic of the treatment criteria.

Could this be better than what we could receive in standard of treatment within our area? And most importantly, was God leading us in this direction? I had specifically asked Him to show us exactly what we needed to do to help Jim through this, and I was willing to pursue anything He directed us to. *Wasn't it worth the extra effort to research this place further?*

If we were going to do it, we needed to work quickly before we started treatment locally. Also, we had no time to waste. The tumor was growing rapidly every day!

In pondering all this, I began to think about who we had contact with in Oklahoma who might have heard anything about this new facility. One of Jim's supervisors from a previous job had moved to Edmond, Oklahoma. a couple of years ago. We were longtime friends with his entire family. In fact, Jim's very best friend and neighbor just happened to be a brother to this man. I felt good about asking him. He was a smart man who would give us sound advice or would go check it out if he didn't know about the place.

When I called and told him what we were facing, I asked him if he had heard of the facility. To my surprise, he told me the center was only a few miles from his home, and he had attended the opening the year before. He was totally impressed with the entire idea and definitely thought it would be worth checking out. Hanging up from my conversation with him, I began to get excited. There are no coincidences with God, and this was beginning to seem like a change in direction for us.

That very day, I called the facility and talked to an inpatient coordinator, who was the friendliest and nicest medical person I had ever visited with. She talked to me for a very long time and answered the myriad of questions I had for her. I expected her to end the conversation by telling me she would send us a brochure on the facility, but instead she asked if it would be okay for a doctor to call me back and discuss the possibilities of whether Jim would be a good candidate for the treatment. She assured me he would tell us very specifically if he believed he was not. He wouldn't waste our precious time. I really liked the sound of that!

Sure enough, the phone rang promptly at 7:00 p.m. The doctor spoke with me for several minutes about Jim's prognosis, and was especially excited to hear he was so recently diagnosed. He asked if I could overnight the disk of Jim's tumor plus the written diagnosis and lab reports so he could make a decision to see if Jim would be a good candidate for their treatment.

I told him I would make a call to the hospital the next day and would be waiting to hear back. Everything I experienced with this opportunity was so positive up to this point! I began to believe something big was going to happen. Hope poured through my body, but I rapidly had to check myself a little. My husband still had inoperable malignant brain cancer! But, again, my God still performed miracles. *Was he about to show us one?*

The next morning, I called the records department of the hospital where the biopsy was performed. I requested they send a copy of the MRI containing the visual of the tumor, plus all lab results, to the treatment center in Oklahoma to the attention of the doctor I had spoken with. I hoped they would be prompt in the delivery and I would hear back from the doctor soon. We were in a race against time. He had emphasized how important it was to begin treatment as soon as possible to ensure greater results.

I kept getting a visual of those horrible cancer cells multiplying inside my husband's brain. But even in the moments of panic, there was an underlying sense of peace that began to take control of my being. I knew and believed the God I trusted was capable of creating answers out of hopelessness. I saw Him begin to open doors I could not have opened on my own.

I felt like I was holding my breath for the next few days as I waited to hear back about the possibility of Jim's candidacy for the new treatment. I received confirmation they had received the medical data and the doctor was reviewing it.

In the meantime, our youngest son Josh had arrived to spend a few days with us. It was so wonderful to have the loving support of our children as we went through these first few days of shock and anxiety. With the chemo appointment only a couple of days away, we really needed to hear back from the treatment center in Oklahoma.

The day before our appointment with the oncologist in Albuquerque, we got the call we had been waiting for. The doctor was optimistic about us coming there for treatment. He felt they could dramatically reduce the tumor successfully and keep Jim's quality of life for a longer period of time. One of the most positive factors was the recent diagnosis of the tumor; also, the fact Jim was very healthy otherwise. Although the facility had mostly treated prostate cancer, one of the most common cancers, they had treated a few brain cancer patients also.

He was very anxious to meet with us and examine Jim in person. I explained we were meeting with an oncologist the next day, and he said it was imperative the doctor give us a referral to the treatment center. He even gave us his personal phone number in case the oncologist had questions about any aspect of the treatment. I knew we had our answer, and I went to bed that night feeling a sense of calmness wash over my whole mind, body, and soul.

As my family and I walked into the oncologist office the next morning, I felt prepared and determined. The young, blond doctor who briskly walked into the room holding Jim's file was a bit of a surprise. She began by explaining what role the oncology department plays in the treatment of the tumor. She wanted to immediately order all kinds of blood work prior to the first chemo. She approached the session in a very business-like manner. I knew I had to jump in quickly before she got any further.

"We understand the treatment philosophy of standard care for this cancer here in Albuquerque. We have researched all the available options, and of course want the very best treatment we can possibly get. We realize no matter what treatment is done, the fact remains that we will only have a limited time. The priority for us is to see Jim's quality of life remain the best it can be for as long as possible. In our research, we came across a treatment center in Oklahoma we would like to pursue. We realize in order to move forward, we need to have a referral from you to assure our insurance will cover it."

She probably had not been with the network of medical doctors and hospitals associated with our insurance company for very long. She seemed uncertain as to how to respond, but she could see the glint of determination in my eye. She began to question what kind of place I was talking about, and as I explained it to her, she wasn't familiar at all with what I was telling her. She mentioned she had occasionally referred patients to another well-known cancer treatment center in Texas, but she knew nothing about the one I was speaking of. I reached in my pocket and pulled out the slip of paper with the doctor's name and number on it.

"Would you be willing to call and talk to a doctor there? He is waiting to answer any questions you might have about this place."

She stood there for a moment, and I could tell she didn't want to make the call. She needed to be loyal to her network.

I looked straight into her eyes. "All right, I will see if I can reach him."

The four of us sat there in a waiting game. My boys and Jim made quiet talk and I fervently prayed. After about twenty minutes, she walked back into the room. Her demeanor had slightly changed.

She looked directly at Jim and asked him pointedly, "Jim, is this other treatment something you want to pursue? I've heard from your wife, but I'd like to hear what you would like to do."

All eyes turned to see Jim's response.

"I want to go where they can give me the best treatment possible that gives me the least damage during the treatments. Yes, I'd like to go there."

Always a man of few words, but he'd said it all.

"Well, I can tell you won't be satisfied here, and you have your minds set on this. The doctor has told me he feels you would be a good candidate since the tumor is newly discovered and you are still in good health. I will agree to grant you the referral."

I could tell she still had loyalty issues, but she must have been somewhat impressed with the doctor on the phone to change her mind. She told us to go ahead and go to the lab for the extensive blood workup. They could send the results over to the new clinic. After the labs, we assumed we would walk out with a referral paper, but the girl at the front desk told us the doctor had already left for lunch and had not left the paperwork for us. We would need to call back when we knew the date that we would see the doctor in Oklahoma. Although this made me a little uneasy, we had gotten her approval and she could fax the referral to the new place. As we drove back home, there was a sense of accomplishment and a sigh of relief that the first big hurdle was over.

After returning home, I quickly punched in the number for the center in Oklahoma. The admitting representative was as excited as we were. She had exuded a sense of personal compassion from the first conversation I had with her a few days earlier.

"How soon can you come? As soon as you tell me the date, I will set up appointments with the radiologist and the oncologist whose office is right next door to our facility."

Suddenly, there were a ton of details to be worked out. The doctor had already told me we would need to plan on being there on an outpatient basis for over two months. Were there places to stay while we were in town that would be both comfortable and affordable? What would we do with our two dogs? Would our home be safe while we were away? Most importantly, would we even have a job when we returned, and would our bosses understand? All aspects we had not even considered until right this moment when the journey became real. We were being thrown into totally unchartered waters and the shock of the cold water hit fast and hard. Another big, red-letter, crisis of faith day. If we truly believed the Lord had led us to this point, wouldn't He provide the answers and direction?

Immediately, He said a resounding YES! Jim had called his best friend back in Kansas and told him we had decided to go to Oklahoma for the treatment. Within a few hours of the call, we received an email from the brother offering to let us stay in their home during the entire time of the treatment. They had a summer home in Colorado they would be going to within the next few days, and their son would meet us in town with the house key and a tour of their home.

We would only be about fifteen minutes from the treatment center, and the route would be light on traffic. We would be coming to the treatment center on back roads from their housing addition in the country. Their home would be our home for however long we needed. This first provision was beyond our wildest dreams!

The dogs would go home with our son, and he would stay at the farm for as long as he possibly could to help get the alfalfa cuttings done. What a relief to my husband, who knew he could totally count on his son to get the work done almost as well as he personally could have done it. He had trained him well all those years as he grew up right by his side from the time he was a toddler riding on the tractors with his dad. His job as an athletic trainer allowed him a few weeks off during the summer, and his very understanding coaches even extended the time for as long as possible. Another unexpected answer to prayer!

Now, for the biggest obstacle. Jim had already talked to his bosses about what had been transpiring in our quickly-changing lives the last few days. They had been very understanding, but also, naturally, extremely concerned. They had thousands of acres of farmland that didn't take care of itself and thousands of dairy cows that got very hungry every day. They depended on top quality corn and alfalfa to fill their bellies to enable them to give productive quantities of milk.

As the day approached for us to leave, we met together here and there with our many Christian friends and neighbors who stopped by with best wishes and times of prayer. Our dear friends, Don and Carita, had invited us over on the Sunday afternoon before we left. They had a friend visiting them over the weekend, and had told us how, as a pastor, he had prayed with many people for physical healing.

As we sat in our friends' living room, the pastor gave us some very wise words. He told us he would pray for Jim's complete healing, but it would be up to the Lord whether the healing would be physical or spiritual. The physical could be complete healing of the cancer and give Jim many more years on this earth. The spiritual could mean the body would die, but Jim would experience complete healing in heaven. It was God's 'perfect will' he would be praying for. We left their home surrounded with a newfound state of peace.

The Friday before we left, I got a call from our intake coordinator at the treatment center saying they still had not received the referral from the oncologist. Odd, as I had notified the doctor's office concerning when our new appointments were and stated we would be needing the referral sent there at once. I again made a quick call, and the office manager said she would put a note in front of the doctor to remind her. An hour passed, and again a call from the Oklahoma office. Still no referral.

The office in Oklahoma was an hour later than New Mexico time. They were willing to wait until 6:00 p.m. in case the doctor needed to wait until all her patients were seen in order to have time to write out the form. A few minutes before 6:00, the Oklahoma office called to get the number of the New Mexico office to talk to them directly.

Finally, after a couple of tense calls back and forth, I received the good news that the form had been received. Whew, another sigh of relief. Doctors could be exasperating at times.

As we packed to leave, butterflies swirled around crazily in my stomach. Even after our insurance paid their part of the treatment costs, we would still have a large sum of money to pay out of our own pockets. But when it came to receiving the best possible care for my husband, money really didn't matter. We had managed to become debt-free in the past few years and might now face a large medical debt. So be it. Situations like this had happened to many others, and we would deal with it the best we could when the time came. Right now, we just had to focus on getting through this.

Chapter 12
The Season of Miracles

June 29, 2010

OUR BOSSES HAD ASKED US TO STOP by their office at the dairy on our way out of town. We would make the stop brief, as we had many long hours to drive. We prayed they hadn't called us in to tell us we had been replaced already, although we wouldn't have blamed them if they did. Our future was so uncertain. We had no idea how Jim would feel after this long ordeal of treatment was over.

As we entered the office, I tried to read their demeanor as they cheerfully greeted us. Not a clue on their faces.

Jim had already told his boss our son had agreed to stay on as long as possible throughout the summer to help in the hay fields. Notes and information had been written out about every possible scenario Jim could think of, and we were always able to be reached by cell phone with questions. There was not much left to say.

Our boss cleared his throat.

"We have been thinking about this for a long time. Even though there is nothing in your contract with us about a retirement plan, we had already decided when the day came for you to retire, we were going to give you a certain amount of money. And it's a pretty significant amount. But under the circumstances, it seems like you might be needing it now. So, here's the first check, and we'll get the rest to you later. Oh, and we will continue to pay your salary while you're gone. Don't worry about any of this while you are away. Just concentrate on what needs to be done. We will see you in a couple of months."

We were too stunned for words! What had just happened? Only the biggest miracle I could ever imagine. In the agriculture industry, farm labor jobs just did not come with a retirement plan. My husband had worked in this area all his life, and unless the farm was a corporation, we had never heard of an individual family farm owner offering any kind of 401K or retirement plan. This was the main reason we had planned to work for at least another ten years to be able to save enough to live during our later years.

Furthermore, although we knew we had given our best in this job, our bosses were not the most demonstrative people when it came to compliments. We felt we had earned their trust since they were spending more and more time away and leaving their place in our responsibility, but never in a million years did we expect to receive this type of generosity—especially with the uncertainty of our future!

I had read and heard of people receiving miracles ever since becoming a Christian all those years ago. I had heard such phrases as "you can't out-give God" and "God provides for His own." I had read Scripture about how generous our Father is in giving good gifts to His children. But in all my life, I had never experienced such an outright, full-blown, bonafide miracle!

Needless to say, we went down the road to Oklahoma rejoicing and more sure of our direction than ever. We had no idea where this new life we were now living was going, or what new twists and turns awaited us, but our faith was renewed and expanded that day like never before.

Several hours later, we were again blessed beyond our wildest dreams! Our friend's son had met us in town, and we had followed him out to the housing edition in the country which contained his parents' home. As we walked through the front door and were led on a tour of all the rooms, we could hardly believe this would be our place of comfort and retreat for the next few weeks.

Spacious and beautifully decorated in rich colors and style, we knew this was another example of how generous our heavenly Father could be. There was a cozy movie room on the top floor with a big screen, and the extra bedrooms and baths would enable members of our family to be able to come visit us on weekends.

There was even a community swimming pool we could enjoy on the hot summer afternoons, and we could take our grandchildren there when they came to see us. We were told over and over again to make ourselves at home while we were there. Our hosts had left a list of their favorite restaurants and stores, and a map showing directions from the house to the treatment center.

That night, after we unpacked our suitcases, we fervently sent up prayers of thankfulness for all the blessings we had received in the course of a few hours. As we fell asleep, we felt encased in the arms of a loving Father who cared abundantly for His children.

The next day being Sunday, we rested and leisurely acquainted ourselves with the house and neighborhood. We drove the few miles on blacktop roads on the route we would be taking every day to the treatment center—roads we would soon be very familiar with. We found the grocery store our friend had penciled in on his map and bought a few items to stock the kitchen where I would be preparing most of our meals.

On the way back to the house, we passed a church on the outskirts of town that piqued our interest. *Would this be the one we should attend while we were here?* We prayed the Lord would direct us to the one that would give us spiritual food during this time of need. As we lay our heads down to sleep that night, again we prayed for specific direction and guidance as we anticipated the doctor appointments the next day and all the long days of therapy in the days ahead.

The sign on the new building stood out in large letters as we drove into the large parking lot the next morning: [1]Procure Proton Therapy Center. Although I had been duly impressed with the friendliness and efficiency of both the initial contact person and the doctor I had spoken with on the phone, I was still unprepared for the reception we received as we walked through the front doors.

We were immediately greeted with warm welcoming smiles and friendly conversation by the two receptionists at the long front desk. "How was your trip? Come around and let us show you how to help yourselves to the various flavored coffee pods, snacks, and fruits laid out on platters. We are so very glad to see you and will do our best to make your time with us as comfortable as possible. Let us set up a time for you to tour the facilities and show you the whole concept of our treatment machines.

"Here is a list of dates and times and addresses of restaurants for our weekly get-together with other patients and staff you are welcome to attend and share a meal with to make your time away from home as enjoyable as possible. While you are waiting for your first appointment with your doctor, have a seat in the comfortable pods with TVs and recliners and book racks. Is there anything else you would like at this time? Your doctor will be out to meet you in the next few minutes."

---

[1] *The new name of the facility is Oklahoma Proton Center. For further information, go to procure.com*

Wait a minute, did they say doctor? We looked at each other, shook our heads in disbelief, and smiled. Then we walked over to the snack bar. I was thinking to myself how this should be the way every medical facility operates: treating their patients as a person, not a number.

Chapter 13
The Painful Thorn

I WISH I COULD SAY THE REST of our day was a continuation of one blessing following another. But hey, we are still living on an imperfect planet with Satan and all his terrible demons running around trying to thwart our good plans and scattering confusion wherever possible.

We are in a constant battle down here where Good and Evil clash and wrestle for the victory, and we must recognize clearly when the battle lines are drawn. We must put on the whole armor of God and prepare ourselves to stand strong with the Lord's mighty power, and never give up. And sometimes it's better not to know just how long and difficult the battle may be, but to fully rely on His strength for the day at hand. These are words of wisdom only gained after living through one of the toughest battles I have ever encountered.

It began after our initial visit with our main doctor, who was as friendly and compassionate as his receptionists had been. He optimistically outlined his strategy for Jim's treatment, which would begin with the construction of a special mask tailor-made to fit his entire head. It would be cast out of a special material that would protect all the rest of the face and brain, allowing the proton beams to only penetrate through the brain to the tumor itself.

Every day, Monday through Friday, we would come to the center, and Jim would spend about thirty minutes receiving the treatments for the next several weeks. Then, midway through the treatments, another MRI would be given to determine how much progress had been done and how many more treatments he would need.

We had already begun the prescription of steroids to keep his body strong and resistant to infection or illness of any kind. He again emphasized how important it was that Jim was still strong and healthy and the diagnosis of the tumor was so recent. This gave us an advantage many other patients did not have who had already tried other forms of treatment before coming to ProCure.

He gave us additional informational brochures about the center and discussed the history and philosophy of how it had originated. We felt surer than ever this was the exact place we needed to be.

Next, we walked across the building through a small library, following one of the receptionists to the connecting medical facility with a different name. This building housed a pharmacy, X-ray and MRI units, and various doctors' offices including the oncologist who would be consulting with our radiologist each step of the way.

As we waited to see the doctor in the waiting area by the oncology office, we got our first hint of trouble. After about thirty minutes, the medical receptionist at the window who had taken our insurance card, called us up and told us there seemed to be some problem with our insurance company approving the transaction. I stated that our oncologist had signed and sent the referral right before we left, so there shouldn't be a problem. The lady suggested we make a call to our insurance to clarify this with them, but they would go ahead and have Jim see the oncologist in the meantime. She stated this was with the understanding if the insurance didn't come through, we would be financially responsible.

A little annoyed and rattled, we went into the doctor's office and sat waiting for the doctor to enter. A petite woman walked into the room carrying a file. She introduced herself to us and quickly got down to business. "I have been reviewing the file ProCure provided to me with all the pathology reports concerning your condition. Has a doctor thoroughly explained the nature of your brain tumor?"

When we indicated we were fully aware of the results, she took a deep breath and looked at us directly. "I want you to understand completely that your tumor is inoperable and growing rapidly. Although ProCure has had some impressive results, the fact is your condition is terminal. The cost of the treatment here will be much more extensive than if you had stayed in Albuquerque and obtained the standard care there.

"Our office personnel have told me there is a question as to whether your insurance is going to agree to pay for this. In my experience with patients with this type of cancer, there may not be much difference in the results time-wise. I just feel like I would be doing you a disservice in not pointing out these facts to you. You will be spending months away from your home and family. If you decide to proceed, I will be willing to work together with your doctor at ProCure in treating the oncology part of your treatment. With a brain tumor, the chemo will be administered in pill form instead of intravenously."

Although others might have been discouraged by her words, I found her honesty completely refreshing. "We have already weighed the options before we got here. We did not come with the errant idea this is a miracle cure. However, we have been convinced Jim's quality of life may be enhanced by choosing this treatment path.

"We live and work in New Mexico, but as far as family goes, we are actually closer to our children here than if we had stayed out there. They will be able to come and visit us more often by coming to Oklahoma. We completely appreciate your straightforward honesty and look forward to seeing you in the coming months."

She shook our hands and wrote out the prescription for the drug called Temodar.

Day one was complete, and we were ready to return to our beautiful place of retreat, so generously provided for us. We were hungry and Jim was tired. When we got back to the house, I would make a quick call to our insurance company and nip the problem in the bud. I was sure there was just a lack of communication and it would be straightened out before any more wrinkles popped up. I decided to wait until the following day to get the prescription filled in the pharmacy.

As we passed by the reception desk on our way out of ProCure, we were given appointments for the following day. One was for the custom fitting and measuring for the mask Jim would be using during treatments. The second was with a lady in the insurance department, and the third was with a financial person to go over the detailed figures involved with the treatment. We felt more strongly than ever this was the place we were supposed to be receiving treatment.

The customer service representative who answered the phone at our insurance office did not have a clue about anything concerning our case. I filled her in about the referral and asked her to please contact the oncologist who had given it to us. I explained where we were and why we were here. She took down our information and I hung up hoping this would be the end of the little glitch of miscommunication.

The next day was busy as we went to each of our three appointments. Jim looked weary as he came out of the doors from the back part of the large complex. He had to lie still for an extended period of time while the mask was molded to his exact head measurements. After the molding dried and the rest of it was constructed, he would return to make sure it fit him perfectly.

For appointment number two, we were led over to a small office just to the right of the receptionist area and introduced to a friendly smiling woman whom I was drawn to immediately. She had the daunting job of dealing with all the various patients' insurance needs. As we sat and chatted with her, I realized she had been one of the people who had stayed late at the office when we were waiting for the referral to be faxed. I told her about the small problem from the day before and asked her if I could get a copy of the referral in case we needed it for future reference.

Peggy explained in general about some of the companies she had dealt with and which ones were more cooperative about approving coverage for the patients here at their facility. She told us to contact her if we had any further issues with our company and she would do everything she could to help. As we left her office, the girls out front remarked that Peggy had been able to accomplish some pretty awesome victories for other patients, and we were in good hands if we needed any help.

Then finally, we went up to the financial affairs office where the man went over all the estimated figures concerning expenses for the treatments. Of course, the final total would depend on how many treatments Jim would ultimately receive, pending the outcome of the MRI at the half-way point.

As a goodwill gesture, we were asked to write out a check for approximately eighty percent of the estimate, which would be held in the safe until the insurance payment was received. As I sat there writing out the check, my hands were shaking. It was the largest amount I had ever written on a check!

In that moment I thanked God, realizing if all else failed and the insurance didn't pay one penny for the treatment, our employers' tremendous generosity meant we would have enough money in the bank to cover it. What would we have done if that money had not been given to us? The realization that at this point we might have had to turn around and gone right back to New Mexico hit me like a brick wall. This was a defining moment when I knew just how much God's provision meant. And I also realized, if it came down to it, I would gladly spend every dollar to ensure my husband got the best.

We walked across the building once more to the pharmacy to fill the prescription for the chemo. As the pharmacist took our insurance card, I literally held my breath as he entered the information into the computer. We sat down and waited while he filled the bottle with the large white pills. There was not another customer in sight, and he began to explain to us how the medication was to be taken.

Then, just as I thought I had had about all the dollar shock I could stand for one day, he told us to handle the bottle with care as we would be holding a prescription worth its weight in gold. He commented that if we had to pay for it in cash, we would be forking out a mere $10,000. Jim nervously laughed, and I about swallowed my tongue. I really thought he must be joking, but when the printout was handed to us along with the pills, the figure was right there in black-and-white. Thankfully, the insurance went through without a hitch.

As we walked outside into the scorching June afternoon, we were ready to sit down in the restaurant across the highway, sip some very cold iced tea, eat a good meal, and let all the events of the day soak in. We talked about the enormity of our endeavor. So much had been thrown at us in such a short period of time. We had really not had a chance to slow down and take it all in.

After all, the rapid chain of events had only begun less than three weeks ago. We drove back to the house, stepped into the cool confines of our new home, changed into some comfy clothes, and lay down for a nap in the dark, quiet bedroom. I didn't know if I could shut my mind down to sleep, but before I knew it, I was waking up to the realization that about five hours had blissfully passed. I felt rested, secure, and completely at peace.

An MRI was scheduled for the following day back at the medical building next door to ProCure. Although Jim had already had the initial one in Albuquerque that first revealed the tumor, this one was not for diagnosis. Its purpose was to gather images of the tumor and normal tissue from many angles for the doctor and other technicians to see the tumor's exact location, size, and shape to enable them to create a personalized treatment plan. It would provide the details necessary for the exact dose of protons needed to precisely target the tumor.

After taking the images, a team of therapy experts would analyze the MRI to determine how many treatments would be needed, the correct dosage of protons, along with which type of treatment room to use. This process of planning could take a few days to complete, after which we would be given an exact schedule of treatment sessions. Finally, another step toward actual treatment was completed. It was exhausting, and we were so relieved when it was finished.

The next day we were ready to relax. There were no appointments scheduled and we badly needed a break. The weather man's forecast was monotonous. The short-term called for record high temperatures. The long-term prediction indicated this could be one of the hottest summers Oklahoma City had seen in years.

After a leisurely breakfast, I decided to take care of a few shopping items I had decided we needed. Although I suggested Jim should stay in the cool house and rest, he wanted to venture out with me and get familiar with some more of the city. Although it was unspoken between us, I had done all the driving since we had first gone to the hospital in Albuquerque. I knew Jim was still more than capable of operating a vehicle, but the raw truth was that there was a cancerous tumor growing inside of his brain. It had already caused one very frightening incident, and we had to face the fact it could happen again.

I am and never will be a confident city driver, being the country girl I'd been all my life. It was just another area I had to hand over to the Lord. He would have to give me an extra sense of direction, quick reaction time, and most of all, guts. It was one more item on my growing prayer list I desperately needed help with.

We had decided to open a post office box since we were unsure of the length of time we would be staying. This would avoid the confusion and extra time of mail being forwarded from New Mexico.

With this accomplished, we headed to an electronics store to make a purchase we felt we needed to keep in touch with our family and friends. It would also afford us the portability we would need during the time we spent in the treatment center. The first iPad had recently come out and it seemed to fit our needs. This would give me an opportunity to keep everyone updated throughout the summer on Jim's progress and provide the tool of research at my fingertips. It would also help me pass the time while Jim was getting his daily treatments.

Another stop at a discount store for a file, hole punch, 3-ring notebook, and notepads, and we were headed back to the house. I found if I kept all the stores and places to stop in perspective to one main street we traveled on most of the way, I could maintain my bearings and sense of direction. As we drove along that main street, I glanced over and saw a sign above a store with a cross on top.

I asked Jim if he felt up to making one last stop before we got home. I hurried into the Christian book store, leaving him in the car with the air conditioner running. This had to be quick, and the funny thing was, I really didn't know for sure what I was looking for. I felt drawn to quickly scan the store for 'something' we could focus on every day during our time here. I asked God to show me what it was. As I skimmed the walls of the last few rows, one plaque jumped out at me. It was a Bible verse in a pretty font with a glassed-in frame surrounding it. I hurriedly pulled it down, walked to the register, and was back in the car in less than ten minutes.

Jim roused from his nap and commented, "That's the fastest shopping I've ever seen you do!"

I laughed and told him I could have easily spent an hour or more in that store, but I knew he was tired and needed to stretch out where he could rest comfortably. He gave me an appreciative look, and I silently thanked God for once again giving me an unselfish heart.

As Jim slept, I went into the beautiful office of our home away from home and began to organize a small area for my use. I pulled out all the papers from the large manila envelope which contained the records from the various medical facilities we had been to in the last few weeks. I wrote out tabs for each doctor or hospital, punched the copies of the physicians' personal notes I had requested before we left New Mexico, and read through each one carefully again.

I looked through the notebook we had received the first day we arrived at ProCure, memorizing each face and names of the doctors, technicians, and other personnel we would be dealing with on a daily basis. I read each page of the description of the history of Proton Therapy and familiarized myself with the medical terminology. Somehow, I knew I was going to have to be smarter and sharper than I had ever been, not even realizing why. But, very soon, I would have the answer, and I would be very grateful I had taken the time to do my homework.

By this time, Jim had been on steroids for over two weeks. The neurologist had explained how they would give his immune system and all other parts of his body a boost, but they also would mess with his sugar levels. As Jim had been dealing with Type 2 Diabetes for many years and had recently gone on insulin, this would mean we would need to keep a close check on his readings.

We had made a pact with each other that every day we were in Oklahoma, we would set aside a special time to read Scripture together, give thanks, and pray for special guidance and healing. We would begin each of these times by reading the words on the plaque I had purchased. It became our claim to ask God to fulfill the promise He had made in those words. We drew strength and faith as we believed His Word is truth.

As Jim was sitting on the side of the bed waiting for me to finish my make-up in the bathroom next door, we had been talking about which Scripture we would begin to study. He had been looking in the back of his Bible at the concordance which grouped subjects by particular words or subjects such as faith, healing, trust, etc. I could glance out the door and see him sitting there as we talked.

One minute he was turning the pages in his Bible, and the next I heard a sudden thud as it hit the floor. As I quickly turned toward him, he gave a slight moan and fell straight back on the bed, his legs still bent with feet on the floor. I rushed into the room and saw that his face was white, and he had gone completely limp!

In a sudden state of panic, I started calling his name and thinking where I had left my cell phone so I could dial 911. But before I could run to find it, he started moving around and coming back to consciousness. I slowly helped him to sit up, get straight on the bed, and lower his body back down. Then I did run to find the phone, call his doctor to discuss what had happened, and figure out what we needed to do.

As quickly as the incident had occurred, it seemed to reverse itself. Jim assured me he was fine, feeling just a little light-headed. After talking to the doctor and getting him to drink some juice and eat a snack, we tested his blood sugar, which was extremely high. The doctor felt the steroids were the culprit but advised me to watch him closely for the rest of the day and let him know if any other symptoms arose. Again, we were reminded how fragile life is and how fast something can happen. How our bodies must be kept in sync and balance, and how just one thing out of order can throw everything out of whack.

After a period of rest, I came back into the bedroom and asked Jim if he felt like having a time of prayer together. I picked up the plaque, and in complete brokenness began to read:

> *Ask, and it will be given to you; seek, and you will find; Knock, and it will be opened to you. For everyone who asks receives, and he who seeks finds, and to him who*

> *knocks it will be opened. Or what man is there among you who, if his son asks for bread, will give him a stone? If you then, being evil, know how to give good gifts to your children, how much more will your Father who is in heaven give good things to those who ask Him.*
>
> —*Matthew 7: 7-9, 11*

With tears flowing freely down my face, I once again placed our lives in His complete control. I asked him to be our Father who would continue to give us what we needed as He had faithfully been doing ever since this nightmare had begun. I asked him to give us the strength, stability, and wisdom to know what to do and how to proceed every day according to His perfect will. I told Him we trusted Him completely and would do whatever He asked, and I meant it with all my heart.

Although the insurance admitted that the young oncologist back in New Mexico had referred us to ProCure, a letter dated July 2 was sent via mail and fax with the following words in bold print: NOTICE OF DENIAL OF MEDICAL COVERAGE. There were several reasons given, but the first was the providers were not part of the provider network. They also had questions about the effectiveness of the treatment, and the consideration that it might be experimental, investigational, or unproven. At the bottom of the letter, we were informed we could file an appeal if we disagreed with their decision.

We would need to fill out the enclosed forms of appeal and within twenty days of receipt of the papers, a decision had to be made by the Plan. If we believed a delay of twenty days might jeopardize our health or life, we could ask for an expedited appeal to shorten the decision time down to seventy-two hours.

A momentary sinking feeling plummeted from my heart down through my stomach as I read through the letter once again. I knew the oncologist had referred other patients to other facilities in other states. She had told us so in her office. The Medical Director at the insurance office was the person who had denied the coverage. Naturally, they would like to keep treatment within the medical network carrying the same name as the insurance company. It made financial sense to do so. *But why would the doctor have written a referral to this place if it was not going to be approved?* I needed to get the answer to that important question before we proceeded.

A frustrating phone call later, during which I was put on hold for about ten minutes while the office manager consulted with the young doctor, (who refused to speak directly with me), brought my blood to a boiling point.

She came back on the line and said, "Although the doctor had written out a referral, it was only for the purpose of consultation at ProCure: to visit the place and see what it was all about, not for actual treatment."

"Did she really think we would be willing to waste the precious time of delaying treatment and absorb all the expense of traveling a long distance to just LOOK at the place? She knew we had already researched the treatment in depth. She took the time to talk on the phone with the director of the facility and returned to us stating she would make the referral. ProCure has a copy of it."

It was obvious she was trying to squirm out of her decision and was attempting to deny it was indeed a legitimate referral.

My next step was a visit to Peggy, the Financial and Insurance Manager at ProCure. As I showed her the letter of refusal, I could tell she was not surprised. This was definitely not her first rodeo with insurance companies.

"I assume you are going to file an appeal," she said as she smiled.

"Well, yes, we have to fight for this. We are Christians, and we gave this matter much prayer before deciding to come here. We felt led to come here, and nothing about this place has changed our minds.

In fact, it has confirmed in every way this is where we are supposed to be."

I looked her straight in the eyes. Her smile only got broader and her eyes shone brightly. "I am a Believer also, so I completely understand where you are coming from. It will take some hard work, time, and effort to fight this, but I will help you through the process. I believe this is the best place for your husband to get treatment, and if you have prayed about it, let's do this together."

God had placed this fine woman here to help us. I knew she was highly skilled to be hired for the position she was in, and I was sure she had helped other countless people. But right at that moment, I understood she was there specifically for us.

The appeal forms were pretty simple, and along with those forms, I composed a personal letter stating our reasons for seeking treatment at ProCure. Jim also signed an Appointment of Personal Representative form allowing me to represent him on the appeal. After composing the letter, I felt sure the refusal would be reversed. The content of the letter follows:

Appeals Division:

I _____, the undersigned, urgently request a reversal of denial for medical treatment at ProCure Proton Therapy Center and _____ Cancer Institute of Oklahoma; _____, Medical Oncology/Hematology; _____, Radiation Oncologist; and any associated medical services for proton therapy.

As documentation will confirm, I was diagnosed with a glioblastoma multiformme (WHO Grade 4) brain tumor after a biopsy was performed by _____, Neurosurgeon on June 14, 2010, at _____, Albuquerque, NM.

After professional consultations with _____, Radiologist, and _____, Hematology Oncologist in Albuquerque June 17, June 21, and June 25, 2010; I was referred by Dr. _____ to

ProCure Proton Therapy Center in Oklahoma City, OK. The referral was made after Dr. _____ conferred via phone for approximately seventeen minutes with _____, Medical Director of ProCure Proton Therapy Center. While my wife, Barbara, and two sons, Chad and Josh, were waiting in Dr. _____ office, she excused herself from the room to make the phone call and to further investigate the best treatment plan. When she returned, she stated to all of us that she was making the referral to the Oklahoma City proton center. We firmly believed that this referral was all we needed to come to Oklahoma for treatment.

We arrived in Oklahoma City on June 29, 2010 and the following day had appointments with the above-mentioned physicians; _____ and _____. As indicated by the physician's notes, they both confirm that proton radiation will result in a much overall better outcome for me, mainly because the radiation will affect 80% less of the healthy cells. Normal x-ray radiation can lead to major side effects, such as balance issues, increased memory loss, etc. as stated by Dr. _____. Especially in brain cancer, side effects to the healthy brain tissue are a major issue. Also, Dr. _____ stated that proton therapy is easier and less stressful to the patient leading to the ability to maintain a more productive lifestyle during the course of treatment itself.

Again, I would like to reiterate that we came to Oklahoma City with the complete understanding that we had received every green light that was required to begin the proton treatment in Oklahoma City.

In addition to the obvious more favorable outcome of receiving proton treatment, the following reasons support the benefits of getting treatment here in Oklahoma City:

- This is the closest city geographically to our home that provides proton therapy.

- It is an FDA approved, non-experimental superior treatment causing less healthy cell damage; particularly important in brain cancer.

- The ProCure Proton Therapy Center has immediate availability, which is crucial to the urgent time factor for starting treatment.

- A home has been provided to us by a close personal friend within fifteen minutes of the therapy center. In New Mexico, the nearest treatment center of any type would be one hour twenty minutes away from our home in heavy traffic across the middle of Albuquerque. This is only for the x-ray type of radiation.

- Oklahoma City is centrally located between our sons who reside in Kansas and Texas. Our third son is currently working at Tinker Air Force Base in Oklahoma City. My wife and I have extended family three hours away in Kansas. From Albuquerque, NM, our closest relatives are nine hours away.

- Our employers have graciously given us the time away from our job to receive full treatment in Oklahoma.

- Our primary care provider, _____, is supportive of my receiving proton radiation and gives her full support and authorization to do so.

In conclusion, in addition to the solid medical facts of the case, I can only appeal personally to ask you to grant me a better opportunity for health and quality of life. As a healthcare provider, much of _____ Plan's literature states that the patient's care and best available treatment is of utmost importance. I implore you to carefully consider the distinct advantage that proton therapy presents to my condition. Mentally I have always and will continue to be a persistent, hard-working individual willing to bravely fight for my very life. I love my children and seven grandchildren, and desire to continue to provide a solid moral and spiritual influence on their lives.

Please do your part to allow this to happen and reconsider your decision to deny me treatment. It is primarily in your hands.

Sincerely,

Along with this letter, we sent all the doctor's notes, the lab results, and all associated records. We sent the copy of the referral. We sent a referral that our primary local physician had written.

We also wrote a request for an expedited appeal. Our doctor from ProCure wrote a letter emphasizing how important it was to begin treatment as soon as possible, as the tumor was rapidly growing. In fact, he stated that proton beam irradiation along with concurrent temozolomide needed to begin immediately in order to halt progression before Jim started developing other neurologic deficits which are usually irreversible once they occur.

As we waited to hear back from the insurance company, ProCure was proceeding with the treatment plan, and finishing the work on the mask that Jim would be wearing during his proton treatments. In the meantime, we were being faithful to our time with the Lord every day, beginning with the reading of the words on the plaque, and studying the Scriptures concerning the subject of faith. Finally, we would pray for each person who would be involved in Jim's care; the doctors, nurses, technicians, Peggy, and yes, especially the people back in Las Cruces who would make the big decisions on our insurance case.

We made an appointment with a natural nutritionalist in Tulsa, who we hoped would provide us with the best nutrition plan to boost Jim's body during this stressful time of battling the cancer. We looked forward to the next weekend when family members were arriving to spend time with us. Although Jim wanted to call back to the farm and check up on the progress and problems that might be occurring, I reminded him that his son was taking care of everything, and right now we needed to focus on our battle right here.

Surprisingly, it became easier for him to do this as the days went by, mainly because of his trust in his son's abilities and decision-making skills he had taught him down through the years.

In two days, we received a reply to our request for the expedited appeal. It stated it had been denied because it failed to meet the requirements under current guidelines. The Medical Director would review the appeal itself and send a decision on it by 08/03/10. If we were not satisfied with the decision of the Medical Director, we could then request an Internal Medical Panel Review made up of appeal reviewers who were not involved in any previous review of our issue.

It is hard to describe how I felt as I read the rejection of our request for the expedited appeal. If our case did not meet their criteria, then what case would? What if ProCure decided to hold up beginning the treatments until the insurance decided to act? I kept thinking how the person who made the decision would feel if it were their spouse whose brain contained a fast-growing tumor.

Chapter 14
The Unexpected Helper

Early July, 2010

AT THIS TIME, GOD AGAIN decided to show us we should persevere. Just when the discouragement and stress threatened to overtake us, another piece of the puzzle fell into place. Our friends, who owned the home we were staying in, had to come back to Oklahoma to attend to a business matter. They were only going to be there for a couple of days. While there in the house with us, we shared about our growing concern and struggles with the insurance company.

The second evening after their return, their son and daughter-in-law dropped by to visit. We knew they were both attorneys but had no idea what their field of expertise was. As we all sat around and chatted, our friend brought up the problems we were experiencing. Listening intently, the woman lawyer began asking me specific questions pertaining to the process. I told her in detail what had happened so far, and after several moments of discussion, she thoughtfully spoke.

"My husband and I deal with specific areas of law. My practice is family law, and my husband deals in another area. But I went to law school with a guy who I think has had some experience in medical law. I've not been in touch with him for a while, but I know he has an office right downtown. I won't promise you anything, but I would be willing to give him a call and see if he could possibly help you out. The last thing you need to be doing during this time is to take on a big insurance company by yourselves."

"Would you really be willing to do this for us?" I implored. My spirits began to rise at the mere thought of getting some legal advice and assistance.

"I'll call him tomorrow. Like I said, I have no idea how busy he may be, or if he would even be interested in taking the case."

A chance return of our friends, and a visit from their children at the exact time we needed help? I couldn't even begin to take in the love our Father continually showed us in His perfect timing.

I had learned from life experience that the squeaky wheel gets the grease. I had discussed this concept with Peggy at ProCure, and she completely agreed. I decided I would get to be on a first-name basis with several of the people at the insurance company, keeping our case on their front burner. Each time I would call, I would jot down the name of the person I talked to, make a note of their position and title in the company, and make the conversation as polite and personal as possible.

I wanted to become a real, living, breathing human being, and not simply a number. At every opportunity, I explained our needs and situation, discussing what was going on with us that day and expressing how urgent it was that our case get immediate attention.

As I got to know Peggy better, she encouraged me to continue to be optimistic. When I told her about the possibility we might be obtaining a lawyer to help with the case, she became extremely excited.

"I have found most people won't continue with the appeal process, and that is exactly what the insurance companies expect. They wear you down with delays and appeals to the point where your already-stressed minds finally just give up. However, I have also found if you continue the process to the end, there have been some successes. And if we put an attorney to represent you into the mix, it just might do the trick. So, don't give up. I'll be there with you all the way through."

She was the encouragement I needed at that moment to keep trying and believing. The very next day, I got the call from our friends' daughter-in-law saying her attorney friend had agreed to meet with us about our case. She gave me the phone number to make contact and wished us luck. I profusely thanked her for her time and effort on our behalf. Within a few minutes, our appointment was made to go downtown and meet with him the very next day. How often does that happen—obtaining an appointment with a busy uptown lawyer within a day? It was a miracle in itself!

The young man who stepped out of his office to greet us was friendly in a subdued sort of way. He began by telling us that although he had taken a few medical cases early on in his practice, he had quickly moved away from that area after experiencing the difficulties and complications they entailed. It was his experience that hospitals, physicians, and insurance companies hire specialized big-time law firms exclusively dealing in these cases, and they were very difficult to go up against. But, because his friend had asked him to help, he would review our case and see if he could be of any assistance to us.

Maybe he wasn't enthusiastically taking our case, but I was grateful anyway. I asked God to give this young man wisdom to help us, and as I opened my file and went through the facts and paperwork up to this point, I tried to impart just how important his help could be. He had his secretary make copies of all the documents and stated his first step would be to request much more information from the insurance company, including our specific policy. He would draft a letter to them informing them he was representing us and strongly encouraging them to grant our petition and fax him the documentation he needed. We left his office with a great sense of relief and hope, profusely expressing our thanks for giving us his precious time and services.

As we soon found out, we certainly needed the services of the attorney who had agreed to take on our case. On July 22, a letter was faxed to ProCure and later received by us via mail stating the Medical Director had decided to uphold the original denial for proton beam therapy. Our appeal was turned down, and our next step was the right to request an Internal Panel Review, which would consist of persons not involved in previous decisions regarding the requested services.

The panel would include seven people, (most of them staff of the insurance company), at least one health care professional specializing in the treatment of the condition being dealt with not attached to the insurance network, and a presiding chairperson of the panel, who would not have voting privileges.

At this appeal, our case would be reviewed, questions would be asked by both sides, supporting material could be submitted up to one day before the hearing, and our case could be presented with the assistance of legal representation. Although we were not surprised at the denial, it meant plainly the battle would have to continue, taking up both time and energy needed to be channeled in another direction. I continually leaned on my faith to provide the sustenance for each and every day.

As I walked into Peggy's office to discuss this new development, something even larger was looming in my mind. "Will the doctors proceed with the treatments despite the insurance delays? Without knowing the final outcome of the insurance coverage?"

She told me she would address this issue with our doctor as soon as he had free time available. We discussed this next appeal, and I told her it would be next to impossible for us to drive or fly back to New Mexcio for the hearing if it was scheduled during the course of our treatments. There would also be the added expense and scheduling of having our attorney go there. She suggested we try to get them to agree to a phone conference hearing that could be held in a room upstairs in their building. This could be attended by several of the doctors and administrators of ProCure. The call would be heard by everyone in the room though the speakerphone.

We faxed the letter of denial over to our attorney and asked him to call me at his convenience to strategize about how to proceed. The one fact concerning me the most was that the panel would consist of the company's employees who would vote on the decision. It seemed like the odds were stacked against us. Then I reminded myself just WHO was right there in control of the entire outcome, regardless of how it appeared from a human standpoint.

The next day, we got a call to come in to ProCure to meet with our doctor. He informed us the treatment plans were complete and handed us a schedule. He was aware of our situation with our insurance company and had consulted with the administration. They had agreed treatment should not be held up any longer. Regardless of the outcome with the appeal process, Jim would receive treatment from ProCure in a timely manner to begin shrinking the tumor.

There was sincere compassion in his voice as he spoke to us, and once again I sensed this man truly believed that this therapy was the best course of treatment. Thanking him just didn't seem adequate, but it was all I could do. He shook our hands and patted Jim gently on the back before he left.

"Don't worry, these sessions will be quick and painless. Most patients experience no side effects other than a little fatigue. Just rest for a while afterwards, then you can feel free to resume normal activity the rest of the day."

The appeal papers were filed, our attorney was handling the legal portion of the case, and Peggy was helping me to tie up all the other loose ends. There were still continual phone calls and information being exchanged almost daily. But now I felt like I had a team working with me instead of flying solo into the great, complicated, unknown world of insurance.

Chapter 15
The Treatment Journey

Late July, 2010

OUR TREATMENT DAYS BEGAN, and a daily routine was finally established. We had purchased a food juicer on the advice of the nutrition doctor, and I began a regimen of preparing all kinds of healthy nutritional drinks from various fruits and vegetables for breakfast, snacks, and evenings. Jim also took many different supplements in pill form. The process of juicing was time-consuming, but I considered it an additional effort well worth every minute invested. As I drank the juices along with my husband, I could feel the healthy results as well.

After driving to the center each day, I sat in the waiting area while Jim was accompanied back to the treatment room for his daily dose of proton radiations. At first, I quietly worked on my iPad by myself, keeping correspondence flowing to our family and friends across the miles. I had put together a lengthy list of people who were updated on our happenings. As time progressed, the list kept getting longer as more friends near and far found out about Jim's cancer and communicated with us, expressing love and prayers and concern.

As I began to update them regularly, I started sharing a few 'moments of faith' testimonies from our many years together as a family. During the long summer afternoons when it was much too hot to even stick our noses out of the house, I found peace and solace upstairs in the cool, darkened 'theater room,' writing short stories and tributes as Jim napped peacefully in the recliner. It was a great source of therapy, along with a faith-building exercise, as I reflected on the many times our Lord had shown Himself to us throughout all the years we had walked with Him.

Reflection and recollection of the hand of God in our journey cemented my personal faith more and more. The words seemed to tumble out of my mind and onto the screen as I typed without effort. I began to realize that miracles, both small and mighty, had transpired throughout our journey over the years. Maybe we recognize them at the time, but more often than not, we regard them in terms of coincidence or even fate, easily dismissing their importance.

This exercise of actually recording the events in black-and-white produced evidence that couldn't be denied. As the stories of our everyday encounters of faith went out to our friends and family in the form of email, I began to receive comments and responses back. It gave me a special blessing to know the stories were touching the hearts of those who read my personal accounts of faith.

Two of the following seemed to elicit the most response:

O HOLY COW NIGHT

"O, Holy Night! The stars are brightly shining!"

How could I possibly think of this magnificent Christmas song at a time like this? But how could I not, when the bedazzling night sky glittered overhead in such glorious splendor, entirely taking my breath away? Countless stars glistened in the massive expanse of crystal-clear canopy, totally overwhelming the parched farmland below. A benevolent silver spherical orb of a moon shone so brightly we had no need of flashlight on that balmy summer night . . . .

Moooooo! Stomp! Stomp! Mooahhhhhh!!!! Hoofbeats becoming louder and more frantic. More and more obtrusive noises penetrating my slumbering brain.

"Do you hear that?? Oh, NO, they're OUT, and this time it sounds like the whole milk-herd!", came Jim's muffled, tired voice from the pillow beside me.

"Oh no!!! It can't be happening again!" I moaned, even as I knew it was real, and we had to move fast, or those cows would be in the next county.

We were smack dab in the middle of the worst drought this normally-lush valley had experienced in a century. It was a record-breaking dry spell. The feed had come up, grown to a height of about six inches, and dried up to a scorched nothingness. Our constantly-hungry one hundred fifty-two milk cows had run out of groceries, and we couldn't afford the escalated hay prices.

Such is the cycle of farming. Scarcity of product drives up market prices. Decreased food supply and hot, acrid weather conditions drops the production of milk, and less milk to sell means less income to buy the high feed.

In our desperation to keep the operation afloat, we had mowed the bar ditches to give the cows something green to eat. Now they were really getting hungry. The scent of our neighbor's wheat patch had prompted our docile herd of Holsteins to take desperate measures. The old fence in the cow pen we had struggled to constantly repair was no match for a bunch of hungry animals. One brave leader breaking through was all it took to persuade the whole herd the grass is truly greener on the other side.

They tromped past our bedroom window with intense purpose. We threw our clothes and shoes on in haste, checked to make sure the boys were all sound asleep, and raced out the door still half asleep. We couldn't take the time to wake up our eleven-year-old to help, and besides, if our youngest woke up and came looking for us, at least he could be soothed by his older brother. Heavy fatigue had become the normal world we lived in daily; not only from the terrific workload of milking, cleaning out the barn, tending the baby calves, and raising three sons, but also from the constant strain of dwindling finances and never-ending dry weather forecasts. How much longer could we hold on? Even without the drought, we were barely hanging onto the farm by our toenails.

As we both raced to opposite sides of the straining mass, I was overwhelmed by the gorgeous array of stars above. Straining to remain focused on the task ahead, I inwardly marveled at the serene, twinkling scene. God's Marvelous Masterpiece refused to be ignored, despite the chaos taking place all about me. Normally those distant stars looked, well, DISTANT, but tonight they seemed amazingly close. The line from the inspired Christmas song unexpectedly surfaced from some place deep within.

Can you imagine trying to turn that many cows completely around and headed back into an empty corral? It is an almost impossible task with several cowboys on horses, or a few people on four-wheelers. How could two weary souls with nothing but waving arms and desperate shouts do the job?

The beautiful sky was forgotten as we went about our frantic task with dogged determination. The hungry bovines ignored us like pesky flies, only turning in circles and avoiding our moves with small kicks and zig-zags. They rapidly fanned out into the field, hungrily snatching clumps of the tender shoots as they walked. Squeaks of plants being pulled up by their roots filled the stillness of the quiet night air, and the freedom of unfenced boundaries created a new spirit of energy within the cows. They had unbridled control, and we were helpless to turn the situation around! Just when we would succeed in turning a couple of the cows in the right direction, they would suddenly wheel back around on us and dodge out of reach. This futile attempt continued on and on until we were worn to a frazzle!

There comes a moment of desperation that defies description. The straw that breaks the camel's back. The moment one can look back on that becomes frozen in time. It had culminated within me for the last couple of months, as we struggled desperately to work just a little bit more each day, striving to overcome adversity with raw determination.

In that instant between insanity and faith, I instinctively cried out to God with complete abandon! "Help me, God; we need your help RIGHT NOW!"

Afterward, Jim would say I ranted at God for several minutes, shaking my fist at the sky, and totally losing it. I honestly don't remember anything after that first outcry. My behavior was so strange and out-of-character, it stopped him dead in his tracks.! The normally optimistic and rather calm personality of his wife had radically changed in the past few moments. What would happen next??

What happened next cannot be explained by human logic. That night in the middle of a wheat field in southern Oklahoma, Jim and I witnessed a true miracle by the Creator of the Universe! The One who hung all those millions of stars in the brilliant night sky, and Who cared enough to hear the desperate cries of His child.

At that very instant, all one hundred fifty-two of those half-starved milk cows raised their heads, turned around, and proceeded to walk placidly back toward their pen. They simply stopped eating, and, in an orderly procession, ambled back home. Jim sprinted ahead, opened the gate, and watched in utter amazement as they passed by! While he moved quickly to put the fence back up where they had busted through, I followed the last one up to the gate and closed it behind them. After a hasty repair, we walked back to the house in quiet shock.

Just before following Jim across the threshold of our kitchen door, I ducked back outside and gazed wistfully up into that vision of wonderment one last time.

"A thrill of Hope, the weary world rejoices,

For yonder breaks a new and glorious morn,

Fall on your knees

O hear the angels voices,

O Night Divine,

O Night, O Night Divine!" *

* *"O Holy Night", Placide Cappeau, 1847*

MIRACLE OF THE FISH

On top of the meager hill up from the calf barn, the red dirt leveled out to catch a scant measure of rain into a glorified mud puddle we called a 'pond.' It measured maybe fifty feet across and about twelve inches deep on a good day but provided just enough of a good swallow to keep us from having to haul water to the dry cows who spent their R&R time grazing amicably on the lush pasture of grass.

I grew up with that good ole red dirt that stained our scalps after playing 'king of the hill' with my older brother and sister. We would throw fistfuls of clods at each other in order to protect the throne at the top, resulting in a good scolding and a thorough scrubbing from Mom at the end of a carefree summer day. I still recall the metal, round tub placed behind the old wash building to provide privacy for us girls. I also remember struggling to stand still while Mama poured pitchers of cool water over my head to rinse out the dark orange silt . . . .

The murky reddish pool prevented any clear view into the water, but for some mysterious reason, it drew the curiosity of our eleven-year-old boy and his fishing pole.

"Dad, can I go fishing up in the little pond?"

"There's nothin in that pond, Chris. It wouldn't be worth the effort."

Jim had waded out into the middle of the water hole, where buried deep into the mud, a plastic pipe ran underground down the hill to provide water to the calf barn. The water above the ground had actually dried up almost completely a few times, just leaving a boggy mud hole for the cows to wade into.

Once, he had rescued an exhausted milk cow from the sticky sludge after the daily count came up one short. He found her struggling in vain to get those embedded hooves loose of the gooey gumbo. It had taken a rope and some pretty persistent pulling to encourage her to make that last valiant effort bringing her freedom yet again!

For four or five days straight, the boy would bring up the subject with his dad. Why encourage such a fruitless endeavor? He would just wind up with an empty hook and muddy boots, not to count the wasted time, which had become precious in our constant struggle to barely keep our heads above water on that dairy. We were lucky to accomplish half of what needed to be done by the time the sun went down on another interminably exhausting day.

"He's just eleven! You can't expect him to do the work of a grown man! He needs to have time to be a kid and have some fun!" my soft mother's heart would protest.

"It will make him tough," was Jim's favorite reply to similar instances when I felt the guilt. Or, "A little work won't hurt him!" I knew my hard-working husband saw the situation from a drastically different perspective of expectation than most. He was the ever-persistent, survive-on-four-or-five-hours-of-sleep, type of man.

How could it be unreasonable to wake his son up at 4:30 a.m. to go out in the dark, round up the milk cows, and spend the next two hours scooping the feed in the troughs as the herd was milked? After all, he got to spend most of the day sitting at a school desk before it was time to go through the whole process again early that evening.

I continually thanked God our son was so gifted in the intelligence department. He rarely brought home homework or needed to study for the big tests. Otherwise, the struggle between my husband and I would have reached greater proportions. I still thought too much was expected of our little boy for his tender age, but most of the time I

tried to keep my mouth shut on the subject. Jim was under a great deal of stress as it was. No need to add a nagging wife to his big list.

"He keeps asking me to fish in that little mud hole, but there can't be anything in it," Jim mentioned to me in passing one morning as we loaded up the calf bottles in the back of the old truck to take across the road to the noisy, bawling bunch.

"Why not let him try? It will give him a break from the chores," (and give him time to just be a care-free kid for a little while, I finished in my mind).

That afternoon when Chris jumped off the school bus and headed to the barn after quickly changing into his chore clothes and grabbing a peanut-butter and jelly sandwich, I hoped Jim would reconsider.

"Mom, I'm goin' fishing!" came the excited voice that crashed back through the door a few minutes later. He was back out and running across the road with his fishing pole and tackle box before I could even respond. The swinging bobber was visible through the kitchen window all the way up the rising slope across the road as my son raced to toss his line into the murky pool.

I turned back to the monotonous twice-a-day task of whisking out the lumps from the Moorman's Smooth Milk Replacement. It didn't quite live up to its name, both in title and function. "Loaded with all the vitamins and nutrients of cow's fresh milk," the label proclaimed. Although we fed them colostrum for their first couple days of newborn life, switching the babies to artificial powdered replacer was tricky business to those delicate stomachs.

After reading articles and receiving advice from neighboring dairymen, I had devised my own recipe to combat the frequent cases of scours and had gotten some pretty good survival rates with my concoction of Gator Aid, Pepto Bismol, and a weakened-down *formula of the powdered milk. Adding needed electrolytes seemed to do the trick.*

Just as I was lugging the wooden bottle crates out the door, I could hear the shouts of pure, unbridled excitement coming from the direction of the old stanchion milk barn.

"Dad, come look at my fish! You gotta see this!"

A FISH. A REAL fish came out of that dinky puddle? I had to see this!

Jim and I exchanged looks of amazement as he strode out the screen door of the milk room; the aroma of warm, rich milk following close behind. Our gazes rapidly were drawn to the flopping, indignant, large-mouth bass struggling at the end of the taut, bending pole. On the other end, our son beamed with pride and delight at our expressions of shock! That bass had to weigh somewhere around three pounds!

The hopeful joy on my little boy's flushed, shining face said it all!

Dear Lord, Let me never be the one who dashes the hope of the seemingly impossible. Of a young person striving to rise above his circumstances of poverty. Of the young couple who has just discovered their unborn baby has a birth defect but decides to continue the pregnancy. Of a middle-aged man diagnosed with inoperable brain cancer who continues to talk about the approaching corn harvest.

Of a little boy who sticks his fishing pole into a mud hole, and believes he is going to catch a fish.

As I continued to write about real incidences from the memory banks of our decades of family history, I marveled at the number of times our great God had shown Himself to us in both small and mega ways. How could I deny for a minute He was there in this present time of crucial, desperate need?

We were at the treatment center five days a week in the late mornings. As we fell into a routine, I began to notice the same people coming in around the same time we did. As time went on, I began to visit with the spouses of the other patients who were in the comfortable waiting area. I discovered most were there to receive the proton treatments for prostate cancer. They had traveled from all over the United States to come to Oklahoma, and for many, this particular place was only part of their cancer story. Some had already experienced surgery and treatment at other types of medical centers before hearing about ProCure. The success rate with prostate cancer using the protons had been quite impressive.

For some people, this was their last hope. Several people expressed how much they wished they had known about ProCure when they were first diagnosed. I felt a hidden guilty pang of envy for the many patients who would be able to go back to their homes after treatment and resume their normal lives. We wouldn't be as fortunate. I had to constantly remind myself about our reality. We hoped for a short-term extension of time and a higher overall quality of life.

Almost every weekend, we had guests come to stay with us. What a blessing it was to be able to host them in the home we had so generously been provided. Whether it was family or friends, they came from near and far to lend support and comfort to us. We did not realize how many wonderful friends and loved ones we had until those visits began to happen.

We had a mini family reunion dinner with my aunt and cousins living close by. Many friends from the various states we had lived in over the course of our years together connected with us first on email, then by phone, then in person. We felt the love physically, emotionally, and spiritually strengthen our weary souls.as we laughed and reminisced about our years together.

Chapter 16
The Guardian Angel

August 25, 2010

THE APPEAL DATE WAS SET. The insurance company had agreed to allow it to transpire via phone conference from ProCure. Our lawyer, Peggy, our doctor, the other Director of Medicine, and some visiting CEOs would be present with us. We had conferred with our lawyer mostly by phone during the days leading up to the conference. We agreed to meet with him a couple of hours before the set time of the appeal conference call, when he would arrive at ProCure early enough to organize his paperwork and get set up in the conference room.

We had said our prayers the night before and given it all up to our Lord. We knew the only recourse left for us if we lost the battle tomorrow was one last appeal before the New Mexico Insurance Commissioner. Although we prayed we wouldn't have to take that last step, I was determined to go the distance if necessary.

We arrived at the center at the usual time for Jim's daily treatment. We would grab a quick lunch in between the treatment time and the appeal. It was going to be a very long and stressful day! After Jim was taken for treatment, I stepped into Peggy's office to talk.

"Well, are you ready for this?" she asked with a smile. "This is a big day at ProCure as well as for you two. It is the first time we have had a lawyer involved in the process, and if it is successful, it could lead to a real breakthrough for us. Some insurance companies wholeheartedly accept our center and pay without a hitch. But for those few we have had to struggle with, it can be a battle. Besides, through this process, you have become much more than a patient to me. I consider you a friend, and I care about what happens to you. It has been so unfair that you and Jim have had to struggle with this aspect while also dealing with all the factors of the cancer and the treatment."

"It has been unbelievably difficult. But I can tell you one thing for sure. You have made it bearable, and I consider you as my special friend now too. Not only are we compatible in our way of thinking, but I know you and I are here together in accordance with God's plan."

Her smile widened and she reached into the top drawer of her desk.

"I want you to keep this with you when we go upstairs for the conference call. It will be a reminder God is with us today."

I looked down to see what she had placed in my hand. It was a pewter figurine of a guardian angel. Words were not needed. I looked up and smiled into her sparkling eyes and squeezed her hands in thanks. This day was already in God's capable hands. We had nothing to fear, regardless of the outcome.

Our lawyer arrived at ProCure around 1:00 p.m., about two hours before the call was to take place. We went over the schedule of how the appeal would proceed. We discussed how at the end Jim and I would have the opportunity to add whatever comments we would like. As we talked, Peggy entered the room with a huge pile of papers fresh off the fax machine.

"You won't believe this!" she exclaimed. "And it is still printing."

The lawyer started shuffling through the stack. He read for a while and shuffled again. He began handing us a few pages to look through.

"This is unbelievable. It seems there is a last-minute effort to attack our case. Someone has been very busy researching on the internet."

I was skimming the pages quickly as he talked. It seemed someone at the insurance office was printing off some negative conclusions about some clinical trial studies.

I had brought my folder pertaining to the rules and regulations of this appeal. Rules, by the way, set up by the insurance company itself. I had read and reread these rules in the last few days. I pulled the sheet out of the folder and pointed out a section of it as I handed it over to the lawyer.

"It looks to me like what they are trying to pull here isn't allowable."

He grinned and shook his head in agreement. "Yes, right here it states that any evidence or paperwork concerning the appeal has to be presented at least twenty-four hours in advance of the appointed time."

"Well, it looks like somebody has sure wasted a lot of paper," my husband remarked with his usual wit and candor.

It broke the tension a little as we were able to smile and relax a bit. The lawyer went to talk to our doctor, and Jim and I got a cold drink. I showed him the angel Peggy had given me, and he grinned.

"Looks like the Good Lord is watching over us again. Peggy is sure a great person."

"I just know she was placed right here for us in this position. Just for us!" I said. Even though it caused us both to laugh a little, I believed it with all my heart.

That last hour dragged by. I spent most of it going over and over in my mind what I would say at the end when given the opportunity to speak to the panel. It could make a big difference in our lives. It would be the last thing they would hear before hanging up and making up their minds how they would vote.

At last the time came for us to get in the elevator and go up to the conference room. As we entered, it occurred to me how huge a deal this was. There were eight to ten people already seated around the huge oval table with the phone sitting in the center. A couple of the doctors weren't even there yet. I desperately hoped they would be able to be there amidst their hectic schedules.

As the minutes ticked down, I kept glancing nervously at my watch. Just as the phone began to ring, the doctors hastily arrived and took the two empty seats. I felt like I had been holding my breath forever as the receptionist's voice came over the line. The conference call was connected, and it finally began.

The moderator for the insurance company in Las Cruces made the introductions of everyone on their end, and our lawyer did the same for us. I appreciated the strong confidence exuded through his voice. In New Mexico, there were six panel members consisting of various personnel from the insurance company. In addition, there was an independent doctor who had not been associated with our case previously. She was an oncologist with previous experience with brain cancer patients, who would answer questions from both sides in reference to her expertise and knowledge concerning the use and effectiveness of various forms of treatments. This doctor would not have a vote in the decision of our case. Neither would the moderator, except in the case of a tie vote.

Each of the members of the panel had read all the factual information in our file, but none of them had been actively involved in the previous two denials of coverage or appeals. I hoped they would be fair, open-minded, and objective. But my rational line of reasoning kept reminding me the bottom line lay in the one glaring fact that each one of them made their living through the employment with the very insurance company we were trying to hold responsible.

After basic introductions, the director at ProCure was asked to generally explain why it was advantageous for Jim to receive treatment here rather than taking the standard care offered in Albuquerque. At great length, he told the story of Proton conception and emphasized it was neither a new or experimental form of cancer treatment. He explained in great detail how Proton therapy uses protons, (heavy, positively charged atomic particles), instead of the X-rays (photons used in standard radiation therapy).

He explained how protons can be precisely controlled so most of their radiation is deposited directly into the tumor, and less of the radiation affects the healthy tissue in front of the tumor. Virtually none of it affects the healthy tissue behind the tumor, therefore patients experience fewer side effects. In regular radiation, much of the energy is released as the X-rays move through the body to the tumor, and again as they exit the body, damaging the healthy tissue in their path. Depending on the location of the tumor, vital organs such as the brain can be damaged by the X-rays.

Another advantage is that proton therapy also can be used to treat tumors that recur after previous treatment with standard X-ray radiation therapy unable to be treated again with X-rays. Typically, there are no or few side effects from proton therapy. Each session, once the patient is situated, usually only lasts about a minute once the proton beam is on. Thirty-three of these fractions should give the brain cancer patient the best chance of long-term local control and asymptomatic life.

Because the side effects are so minimal, there is less stress for the brain cancer patient, and it will spare the remainder of the brain, which can continue to function normally. With regular radiation treatment, side effects such as balance issues, increased memory loss, and overall fatigue can greatly affect quality of life. Proton therapy will affect an estimated 80% less of healthy cells compared to standard radiation treatment.

"Therefore, there is a great advantage of proceeding with the treatment offered here at ProCure versus the standard care that is the only option back in New Mexico," he concluded.

Next, our personal doctor at ProCure went into detail explaining all the procedures that had taken place since we had arrived several weeks ago in OKC. He again emphasized just how critical it had been to immediately begin the treatment process before other parts of Jim's brain were affected by the growth of the tumor. Because of ProCure's dedication to serving the best interest of the health of the patient, an executive decision had been made by the facility to proceed with the treatments despite the insurance company's hesitancy in confirming coverage.

At that moment, once again I saw our Father's Hand in our journey. How many facilities would have proceeded without the complete guarantee of coverage?

After the initial statements, the panel in Las Cruces could each ask a question or state their opinion. It is amazing how much can be read from a person's tone of voice. The first man to speak came across as no-nonsense, factual, and negative. He not only questioned the authenticity of proton treatment but said that his personal research had led him to conclude the effectiveness of the protons versus standard care treatment was inconclusive. I could tell right away he was probably a no vote. As the most vocal of the panel, he then asked for the panel to review and refer to the huge stack of research he was obviously responsible for. These were the papers that had been faxed to the office a short time before the call.

Immediately, our lawyer jumped into the conversation and pointed out the rules specifically stated all evidence or documents must be received twenty-four hours before the hearing, and since this did not occur, it would have to be dismissed and discarded from discussion in this case. The moderator immediately concurred with this point and told the panel to disregard the evidence.

I silently thanked the Lord for the foresight to see this coming in advance. A few others asked a couple of questions of the doctors and administrators. Although they were more polite, I could tell they also had great reservations about ProCure in general.

Our lawyer then presented his case to the panel based on the research he had done concerning the insurance policy itself, citing the language in various places that referred to the various terms in the rules throughout the document. The biggest issue seemed to boil down to *out of service area* coverage. Although it was not common in practice, he referred to examples where patients had been referred to *out of area medical facilities* for second opinions and treatment.

This was based on specific well-known clinics he had directly contacted to support and confirm this evidence. He read from the policy itself which at times seemed to contradict itself on this point, but which ultimately allowed treatment elsewhere after referral from an in-service physician. He asked the panel to look at the referral given to us by the young oncologist, who initially had talked to the doctor at ProCure, and who finally faxed the referral.

He then went over the evidence of the solid history behind proton therapy and discussed how it was neither an experimental or unproven treatment. He presented the fact that one of the most famous centers for cancer treatment in America had plans to build on a proton treatment machine in their huge conglomeration of buildings to treat certain forms of cancer. This was a big surprise to me, but I was so thankful he had discovered this very important fact. *Surely this would make an impact on the listening panel.*

Finally, the cancer oncologist who was standing by, got on the phone and both sides were able to ask specific questions of her, based on her experience and opinion. She had neither been involved with us or our insurance provider but worked for a university medical facility in Albuquerque. Several questions were asked about the specific kind of cancer Jim had and her experience in treating it personally. She confirmed the type of cancer we were dealing with is one of the most serious and fastest-growing types, and her experience was that most patients survived only a couple of years or less after being diagnosed. After being questioned about her knowledge of proton therapy, and the possible advantages it might produce, she admitted she was thoroughly unfamiliar with it.

A member of the insurance panel asked her if she felt that traveling out of area to pursue an alternative form of treatment would be advised. Our doctor interjected that because she was uninformed about proton therapy, it would be difficult for her to make an informed opinion on this question. Our doctor then proceeded to explain the general principles and processes. The insurance panelist again asked her opinion on the matter.

"Knowing the rapid progression and mortality rate of the particular cancer we are discussing, I would probably encourage the patient to stay put in his comfortable, local environment and receive the standard regimen of treatment."

Without hesitation, our doctor came back with this follow-up question:

"For a moment, let's imagine you or a loved one very close to you was diagnosed with this very form of brain cancer. You lived in a city where on one block a standard radiation medical facility offered treatment that would reduce the tumor for a short period of time. In the process of radiating the tumor, other brain tissue would be affected which could alter certain physical or mental functions. Down the street, a proton radiation facility stood, offering a way to pinpoint the tumor with much more accurate and precise beams, also shrinking the tumor down, but not scattering the rays to other brain tissue. This allows your loved one at least the same or added amount of time to live, but also experiencing a more normal brain function during those remaining months. Which facility would you enter?"

There was a period of silence on the phone that to me, and I hoped to everyone else listening, spoke volumes. I'd always heard the phrase about a 'pregnant pause,' and how silence can speak volumes, but never had I experienced such a moment in my entire life like this one. During the long span of silence, I found myself holding my breath. Everyone sitting around our huge oval table froze in place as not one single movement or sound occurred. I held tighter to Peggy's angel in my hand beneath the table.

"I would have to say that I would need to research the proton history and procedures thoroughly before making a decision. But if I was convinced it could give my loved one a better quality of life, I would pursue that avenue."

On our end of the conversation, everyone seemed to exhale and smile at each other in unison. Our lawyer gave a thumbs-up to Dr. Alex, and I could feel the blood start to pump through my body again.

"But there is no option of a proton facility in the policy holder's area of service," a panel member interjected.

Our lawyer swiftly came back with a reply.

"If it was your loved one, would a few hours away from home make any difference? How far would you go to give your family member the best option of care under these circumstances?"

The call was drawing to a close, and at this point the moderator for the insurance company asked if anyone on either side of the line would like to make a closing statement. At this point, our lawyer looked at Jim and me with a question mark in his eyes.

Although we had just experienced a great moment, I had to do all I could to convince this panel we had the right to be covered by their insurance.

I signaled that I would like to speak. The lawyer introduced me, and I prayed with all my heart I would say the right words:

"I would first like to say we would not be sitting here having this conservation if the oncologist back in Albuquerque had not signed the referral and faxed it to this facility. I would also like to tell you how very difficult and stressful it has been, in addition to the shock of learning about this life-changing, tragic diagnosis, to have had to struggle and fight for our health insurance company to provide us with the coverage to enable Jim to receive the treatment he so urgently requires.

"Since the first day we arrived, in addition to thinking about how to manage each day of surviving this dreadful disease, I have also had to deal with countless hours of phone calls, paperwork, and appeals related to our health coverage. We have had to hire a lawyer. We have had to delay the schedule of the treatments, waiting to hear that we were covered. We have had to agonize over whether to go ahead and proceed with treatment, knowing with each passing day, the tumor in Jim's brain was aggressively growing. We have had to deal with unanswered questions, undeserved negativity, and oftentimes, confusion and inconsistency from your office.

"And all we desire is the best chance, the best option for the short time of life Jim has in front of him. Your literature states that your insurance company always has the health and well-being of the patient at the forefront—that your intention is to always provide the assurance that you are receiving the best medical care available.

"I researched all the options, I did my homework to discover the best route we could take to make these months ahead as painless and positive as they can be for my husband. Knowing our time is short, I had to make the best choices. There is no time to waver or go from one form of therapy to another. In the short time remaining, I would like my husband to have the best quality of life possible. ProCure Proton Therapy Center gives Jim that opportunity over the standard care available in New Mexico. Isn't that what you would do for your loved one in this situation? I asked and plead with you to take this matter down to a personal level. I ask you to make your decision from a human perspective rather than a legalistic one. Thank you in advance for doing the right thing."

I felt drained. I had hung my heart out to these complete strangers. There was nothing more to be done. The moderator announced the panel would now discuss the matter and vote. She would call me within twenty-four hours with their decision.

We got up, shook hands with the lawyer, rode the elevator down to the main floor in silence, and took our leave after saying goodbye to Peggy. I really didn't know what to think. Not once during the whole phone call did anyone on the New Mexico end give one word of compassion or indication they might be voting positively for us. We were exhausted and spent.

We had done all we could do. There was nothing left except the long twenty-four hours ahead of waiting. This whole process had taken its toll on me. I wished I could just be knocked out and awaken to find this whole big mess had been a nightmare. I just wanted to wake up, get dressed, and head out to the green alfalfa fields—to breathe in the smells of nature, take a long walk with Samson down the dirt roads, and watch the gorgeous display of the New Mexico sunsets.

What I wouldn't give to be living the normal, peaceful, everyday farm life once again. As I lay down to sleep that night, more than ever I realized nothing in our lives would be normal for as far ahead as I could imagine.

"Lord, you have to carry us through this uncertainty one day and one decision at a time. You already know what the phone call will tell us tomorrow. I'm counting on You. I'm trusting You with it all. It's much too big for me to carry. I can't even think about it anymore." And with that, I fell into a deep sleep in the beautiful house provided to us as a place of refuge and peace.

Chapter 17
The Day of Decision

The Next Day

THE HOURS DRUG BY AS we waited for the Big Decision the next day. We went about our daily routine on automatic pilot. We got up, drank the tall glass of fruit and vegetable juice I had prepared in the juicer the evening before, ate a nutritious breakfast, showered, and got ready for the daily trip to the center for Jim's treatment. Jim had downed the dozen or so supplement pills to boost his immune system recommended by the natural health doctor in Tulsa.

After treatment, we popped into Peggy's office to let her know the phone call had not come yet. We briefly rehashed the call from the day before, and all agreed the decision could go either way. We were resolved to go to the next level if we lost this appeal, but we also knew our chances of being successful would greatly decrease if we had to pursue that route. With a promise to call her the minute we heard anything, we headed back to the front desk to check out. The girls there gave us an encouraging word and smile, reminding us there would be a 'meal about town' that evening at 6:00 p.m. for patients and staff to fellowship and dine together. They hoped it would be a time for us to celebrate our victory. Oh, how we hoped that would be the case!

Knowing the call would most likely come before 5:00 p.m. Mountain Time, we hoped to receive word sometime during the afternoon hours while we were back at the house. By 4:00 p.m. Central Time, my cell phone had rung twice, both times making me jump with the expectation THE CALL was happening. But the first one was our lawyer checking in to see if we'd gotten any word yet, and the second later in the afternoon from Peggy. By this time, we were both getting extremely nervous and exasperated. If the decision had been made last night, why hadn't they called by now?

I tried to force my mind away from the negative. It was hard not to think about the tone of voice the panel members used. Stiff, uncaring, completely business-like. Fear threatened to overcome my trust. As the clock ticked on, I found myself wanting to just stay home and give into the fear. What if they didn't call today at all? How could I go through another night of waiting for the news that held such power over our future? I wavered between trust in the Lord who had already given us so many powerful signs of His love and control over our situation, and the fear of knowing this decision rested in the hands of human minds who very well could care only about their job security and appearance amidst their peers.

After Jim awoke from a much-needed nap, I decided to leave the decision of whether we would go to the social up to him and how he felt. Without hesitation, he said we should get ready and go.

"It's better than sitting around here waiting for the phone to ring," he flatly stated.

He was right, but my enthusiasm for dining with a group of people and trying to make pleasant conversation was very difficult to muster up. And they would be sure to ask us how our appeal had turned out, as word traveled quickly among our little group about such things.

Knowing we needed to allow a half-hour to find the unfamiliar restaurant, we left the house at 5:30 p.m. Concentrating on the written directions Jim was reading from, my mind became totally focused on the unfamiliar exits and rush hour traffic. I knew the chosen restaurant was out by a lake in the countryside. Once we got away from the main traffic of the city, we were on a rural black-top road with open fields and pastures on both sides. Wild sunflowers filled the ditches, and cattle grazed around a small farm pond. Soaking in the familiar, unexpected rural scenery, I found my taut muscles begin to relax and my breathing slow down. My tight grip on the steering wheel loosened a little. I could also sense Jim begin to relax as he chatted about what might be happening back on the farm in New Mexico.

I thought about how relieved I was that he seemed to be less and less concerned about what problems and big decisions he was missing out on. Knowing how seriously he took his job, I had been afraid he would constantly worry during his absence. I had encouraged our son to keep conversations with his dad brief and optimistic concerning the daily decisions and problems that might be happening back on the farm. At the same time, I emphasized to Jim how important it was to concentrate on his daily progress through treatment, nutrition, and a spiritually positive state of mind. Being physically distanced completely from the farm had worked to separate Jim from the stress. I was again reassured our decision was right.

My thoughts were suddenly interrupted by the sound of my phone ringing in the console between us. I immediately slowed down, looked over at Jim, and reached for the phone. As I pulled over as far as I could on the narrow shoulder and applied the brake, I glanced at the phone screen. The name of the insurance company flashed on the screen.

This was it! As I quickly shoved the gearshift into park, I caught sight of the clock on the car dashboard. 5:55 p.m.

"Hello, is this Mrs. McCune?"

"Yes, it is."

"This is Lesley, calling from _____ Insurance Company in Las Cruces. I was the moderator yesterday on your appeal conference call. I'm calling to tell you the result of your appeal. Can you hear me all right?"

"Yes, I can."

"After the call, there was a lengthy discussion, then votes were cast. As it turned out, there were three votes of yes, and three votes of no. Therefore I, as the moderator, had to cast the vote to break the tie. The ending result is four yeses, and three nos. However, there is a condition on the decision. The insurance company will pay for treatment based on what the standard treatment would have been had you stayed in-area. Whatever expense above that amount will be your responsibility. You will be sent the official written decision, as will your lawyer and Procure Therapy Center, within the next ten days. Do you have any questions?"

I swallowed hard as my mind tried to absorb what she had told me. Our lawyer had told us it was likely, even with a positive outcome, that the insurance company might not be willing to pay with complete coverage the total amount. He told us to keep in mind a "yes" at this point in the available appeal process was a huge victory.

"No, I don't have questions at this point. I will relay this news to our lawyer and if he might have any questions, he can call you. Please give me your full name and phone number, so he can directly talk with you if he needs to. And, one more thing. I know you probably cannot go into detail about how the decision was reached. But I want to personally thank you for the vote you cast. Your vote has enabled us to complete this treatment process with peace of mind and closure. You have no idea how stressful it has been to have had to deal with this issue hanging over our head while at the same time dealing with the shock of the cancer itself. Whatever caused you to vote yes for us,

I can't tell you how much it means to us. It literally changes our lives. I want you to understand that."

The softness in her tone of voice came over the line in her reply.

"I wish you the best. My name is _____ _____, and your lawyer can reach me personally at _____. Have a good evening, Mrs. McCune."

Jim had been watching me closely as I talked. When I put the phone back in the console, tears began to run down my cheeks.

"It came down to a tie-breaker. Three for, and three against. But the moderator, this woman I was talking to, voted for us, and WE WON!"

I then explained the condition they had put on it, but emphasized the important thing was WE WON! I realized as I repeated the news to Jim, I had been prepared for the worst. We had lost two appeals before this. We had been forced to fight even harder. I had made so many calls and talked to so many different people at that agency. I had been put on hold for long lengths of time. I had been shuffled from one department to another, most often talking to a different person whom I would have to explain our situation to over, and over again. I had gotten the runaround and, more often than not, very confusing and uncertain information. The wheels had turned slowly, the attitudes had often been indifferent or brusque, the battle had been long and frustrating.

Would we have won without all the help we received through our lawyer, our caring doctors, and our persistent and loving Peggy? The answer is a resounding NO! Without a doubt. But would I have gone through it all if I had it to do all over again? The answer is a resounding YES! I just had to keep trying until there was no further place to go. I had determined to be persistent and smart, polite, yet forceful. I became convinced the overall strategy of a big company was to make the process as drawn out and complicated as possible, hoping the individual will find it so overwhelming and difficult, they would fold up and quit. I was so thankful I had stuck it out. But I could not have made it without the help and strength of the Lord, who ultimately has control over it all.

We walked into the restaurant after making calls to Peggy and the lawyer to tell them the verdict. Peggy was totally excited and promised she would do what she could to work with her supervisors on the difference between what the insurance agreed to pay and what the total bill would be. Our lawyer was positive and felt like we had gotten the best deal we could have, given the circumstances. By the time we went into the dining area, everyone else who had come with our group was already seated.

One of the girls from the reception desk was at the first table. She immediately asked if we had gotten any news yet. The good news spread quickly throughout the line of tables, and we soon were receiving congratulations from nearly everyone. After such a long expanse of waiting, it felt wonderful to finally sit down and relax.

As we had come in late, it wasn't until after we had eaten that we had a chance to go out the back of the restaurant to catch a breathtaking view of the lake. As the sun set over the water, dark storm clouds suddenly appeared in the western sky. A fast-moving summer storm developed at the far end of the lake, and its narrow path moved swiftly, heading directly toward us. We stood absolutely spellbound by the dramatic effects of lightning bolts and the accelerating rumble of thunder getting closer by the minute. In my entire life, I had never witnessed such a narrow, intense array displayed right before my eyes.

It traveled straight toward us! The water in the direct path of the storm sent waves peaking on both sides as the great accompanying wind furrowed its path. Although it appeared the very spot on which we stood would soon be consumed by its rage, all of us standing on the open deck were paralyzed in the fascination of it all. It was as if our shoes were glued down, and we were powerless to move out of its path. Just as it looked like it would strike us with full force, it suddenly veered off to one side and completely disappeared from our view!

Everyone began to talk animatedly to each other, none of us able to absorb what we had just witnessed.

On the ride home in the car, I could only shake my head in wonder and try to figure out what the meaning of it all was. I believe to this day there was a message given to us in those moments of raw, exciting intensity. Sometimes, when the storm is coming right at you with full force, and there seems to be no escape, the hand of God reaches down and redirects the path, rescuing you at the last possible moment. It was exactly what He had done with our insurance appeal. I will never forget the miracle of that rescue for us—nor the visible object lesson presented vividly to us that very special night on the lake.

My, what a blissful night of sleep we both enjoyed after returning to our peaceful place of retreat that evening. I had not slept so well since the night back on the farm in June before this whole nightmare had begun. We were finally free to settle in and concentrate on the days of treatment ahead. The huge, dark cloud of concern over the financial aspect of our situation was removed. Yes, we still had unbelievably difficult days ahead, but one more tremendous provision had refreshed our faith and enabled us to keep standing.

Chapter 18
The Graduation

Late September, 2010

OUR DAYS FELL INTO A ROUTINE as the immense summer heat continued. Jim would get up, shower, drink a tall glass of prepared vegetable/fruit juice, take a dozen or more vitamin and mineral supplements along with steroids and diabetic insulin shot and pills, and get ready to leave for the treatment center. After the treatment, we would go across the street and eat a low-fat, nutritious meal or go home and fix lunch. We followed lunch with a time of reading our Bible and prayer, then Jim would settle in for a time of rest and a nap. I would have a quiet time to write on my iPad, pay bills, communicate with friends and family, do laundry, and clean.

After a light evening meal and more juice and pills, we would go for a short walk around the neighborhood or a refreshing swim in the community pool depending on what the heat allowed us to do. Jim would then enjoy watching TV or a movie in the comfortable dark theater room upstairs, while I cut, chopped and juiced a whole variety of fresh fruits and vegetables for the following day's supply. On weekends, friends or family would arrive to spend a day or two visiting us. Every Sunday morning, we would drive the few miles to attend the Life Church, bringing along our friends or family members who might be with us.

One very special weekend, all seven of our grandchildren got to be there all at the same time. Because they lived in Nebraska, Kansas, and Texas, we had never had them altogether in one place. It was a blessing beyond measure. We took many pictures of memories treasured that weekend. Grandpa, "Papa" Jim, was on cloud nine as we enjoyed a time together in the pool with him surrounded by his special babies!

No grandparent was prouder of his grandchildren than he was. He was unashamedly one of those Grandpas who would whip out his billfold and tell a special story about one of his brilliant grandsons or granddaughters everywhere he went. His were the brightest, cutest, most special specimens of human beings ever born on this earth. His greatest sorrow was facing the reality he would not be able to see each of those children grow up, graduate, marry, and have babies of their own. We both cherished the weekend with our 'magnificent seven' more than they would ever know.

Another weekend, five of our friends from high school came down to visit for a day from Kansas. It was great to laugh and reminisce for a few hours together. We had visits from relatives and friends whom we had not seen in years and years. Our very close friends and pastor for many years came to see us one day at the treatment center as they were traveling with their daughter and family on a vacation and passing through Oklahoma City on their way.

It seemed like a special, highlighted parade of all the special people who had passed through our lives in all the forty years we had done life together. They arrived from Nebraska, Kansas, Oklahoma, and Texas. Each one encouraged us in their own special way. We realized how important people are. Not our possessions, our jobs, our successes, our bank accounts, but the pure joy of special relationships with family and friends who had touched and enriched our lives down through the years.

As the days and weeks passed by, the end of our time in Oklahoma City was finally drawing to an end. We were told about a 'graduation ceremony' to be held one morning after the completion of the treatment process. We could invite a few special guests to share our celebration time. There would be three or four other people graduating on the same day as Jim. Each graduate would have the opportunity to give a little speech, one of the doctors would speak, and each person would be given a special gold coin to commemorate their time at the center. In the future, when revisiting the center, the coin could be presented to prove your alumni status.

After the ceremony, a reception would be held with family, friends, and whatever treatment center personnel were able to attend. There would even be a special personalized cake in each person's honor. We were overwhelmed with the caring, special celebration being planned just for us!

As the monumental day drew near, the two of us began to plan how we would like to make it memorable. As we began to talk about Jim's speech, we decided to honor not only our family who would be attending, but also one very dear person, without whom we would never have made it through. I was excited to hear what Jim would say. He spent quite a lot of time jotting down an outline, and although I wanted to peek at his words, it needed to totally come from his thoughts and heart.

Finally, the last treatment was over, the house was scrubbed top to bottom, our bags were mostly packed, and we were prepared to leave for home the next morning after the graduation ceremony. My mom and sister and brother-in-law from Kansas were meeting us at the center.

It was bittersweet as we made the final fifteen-minute drive into town. Could it have been three months since our apprehensive trip to a place we had only learned about a few days before we arrived—following the sweet direction of the Lord?

Many emotions washed over us as we arrived at the treatment center that had become almost like a second home to us for a few short months. These doctors, technicians, insurance managers, and receptionists had become our allies and friends. They were our frontline defense workers against this horrid enemy called cancer that had invaded every aspect of our lives. We were here to celebrate this three-month battle. We still had a very uncertain future ahead of us, but this strategic counter-attack had hopefully given us a powerful boost and delay in both time and quality of life for the next few precious months.

The room was charged with an upbeat, positive vibe. Family, friends, doctors, nurses, technicians, and other medical personnel wearing their scrubs were scattered throughout the room. As one of the directors opened the program, we proudly sat among many who had come from all over the country looking for hope and treatment with various types of cancer.

An alumnus came forward and gave his personal success story, praising not only the treatment, but the amazing personal care given to him during his time at ProCure. He drew the gold coin from his pocket, showing the date his graduation had taken place. Four years had passed, and he was still cancer-free from the prostate cancer which had invaded his body.

Several other patients came to the front of the room and shared about their personal experience. Some had been in Oklahoma City for a few weeks, while others like Jim had received approximately two to three months of treatment. The common thread which ran through almost all the testimonies was not only the confidence each had in the facility to treat their cancer, but the most unusual and exceptional personal care they experienced.

I was nervous for Jim as he walked to the front to give his speech. This was not his forte to stand up in front of a crowded room of people to speak. But the sincerity and humbleness of character immediately shone through any nerves he might have had. He briefly summarized how he had found out he had the brain tumor, and the story of our journey that led us to this place. He also praised the doctors and other medical personnel who treated us with such tender loving care, even to the point of placing his life and treatment above our ability to pay the bill or knowing whether our insurance would ultimately come through and cover him. He thanked family and friends and most of all, God, for being his rock though all the upheaval in his life since that fateful day of diagnosis.

"And finally," he said with a smile, "I want to honor one very special lady who went above and beyond to help us out during our stay here. She has a little office over to the side and is oftentimes overlooked. But to us, she was our special angel, never giving up in her efforts to help us fight the big insurance company that basically could make or break us financially with their decision on whether to cover us or not. She worked many long hours with my wife, always encouraging us and giving us wise advice at every step. Without Peggy and the good Lord above, our outcome would no doubt have turned out differently. Peggy, would you come up here? I have something for you." His voice trembled with emotion on the last few words.

As Peggy walked up to stand beside Jim, he reached behind him and handed her a plaque. It was a picture the three of us had taken together a couple of days after we had learned of our victory with the insurance company. Jim and I stood with our arms around Peggy's shoulders, all of us beaming brightly into the camera. There was also a personal note of gratitude. Tears began sliding down Peggy's cheeks as she gave Jim a special hug. All of us in our cluster of family sitting in our row of seats began to cry also. This was a poignant moment of reflection and celebration imprinted indelibly on my memory.

After each graduate received their personal gold coin, everyone celebrated with cake and drinks. Each cake was specially created with the graduate's name and date of graduation. I again marveled at the personal attention to detail given to each person. We chatted with as many personnel as possible to personally thank them for all they had done for us, although many had dashed back to work right after the program.

We did not get the opportunity to express our complete and full gratitude to our main doctor face-to-face, but I vowed within myself to write a personal letter after we got home. I had caught a glimpse of him in the celebration room as he slipped in for a few moments in his doctor's coat, but when it was over, he was gone. I hoped he had been able to stay long enough to hear Jim's heartfelt message.

Without his personal, lengthy phone call with me as I searched out the possibilities of treatment, the decision to proceed with Procure would not have happened. I couldn't imagine another physician taking about twenty minutes of his precious evening time talking to a perfect stranger in another state, patiently explaining and answering my every question. I also knew we would be returning for the follow-up visit in a few months, when another full MRI would be performed to measure the tumor again, and to discuss the results with him.

After a celebratory lunch with our family across the street, we bid them goodbye and went back across to ProCure for one last business detail. We walked up the stairs to the business office and gently knocked on the door.

"We are here to determine how you want to tie up the financial part of our treatment costs. We know Peggy has been in touch with you to keep you informed about our insurance battle and the outcome of our appeal. Do you still want to hold the check we gave you until you receive the funds from them?"

The young man smiled and reached into his top right drawer. "We won't be needing to retain this any longer. If there is a balance after the insurance funds come through, we will send out a bill. I know you must be greatly relieved to be getting this back into your hands."

"You have no idea! Absolutely no idea!" I emphatically exclaimed.

Although I didn't tell him, this money would have made the difference between us having no future options as far as housing and standard of living for the immediate future and being able to have those choices possible. In my wildest dreams, I had not imagined we would ever find ourselves in this extremely vulnerable and desperate place.

I took the check and placed it in my purse. What a visual reminder of how our lives could virtually hang in the balance.

Our last stop was for a quick last hug in Peggy's office. She proudly pointed to the wall across from her desk.

"This will always be a reminder to me to keep fighting and persisting for all the future people who might need my assistance down the road. I'll never forget you and the time we spent together. It's why I work here and do this job."

"Thank goodness you have been given this great gift of persistence and wisdom. Personally, we know God placed you right here just for us at this time," I said, looking into her sweet face.

I knew without a doubt what I had told Peggy was just one more example of God's provision. Again, and again, we had seen it along this journey. Obvious, direct, generous gifts from a merciful and loving Father.

After leaving a lengthy note of gratitude on the kitchen counter for our friends to find when they returned home from Colorado in a few days, we finished loading up the SUV, checked the house thoroughly one more time, and closed the garage door. As always, before departing on a trip, we held hands and prayed for our long drive ahead as we journeyed back to New Mexico.

Stopping to take one long last look at the beautiful home we had the privilege of staying in for the last three months, I shifted the vehicle into drive and gave a big sigh of both satisfaction and apprehension about our next step into the uncertain future. Jim was extremely anxious to return to his farm—finally allowing himself to shift gears from the treatment process to those drying fields of corn awaiting harvest shortly after we returned. The powerful drive at the core of his being began to awaken as the miles rolled by. He was morphing back into the role of farm manager, and I could see him begin to take the huge responsibility squarely back onto his big shoulders.

Chapter 19
The Homecoming

AS I DROVE ACROSS THE OPEN plains of western Oklahoma, and the vast drylands of the Texas Panhandle toward our home, I also began to anticipate the coming harvest awaiting us upon our arrival. We wouldn't have the luxury of long days of rest and recuperation as we transitioned back into our past lives. We would have to immediately hit the ground running into one of the busiest times of the year on the farm.

Timing was everything when it came to the harvest of the corn fields which had grown all summer into thick rows of stalks with loaded ears. Months of sunshine and irrigated water resulted in the bountiful crop that would feed over two thousand head of dairy cattle throughout the coming year. As the stalks dried out to just the right moisture after the watering was shut off, all the machinery was being checked over in the large machine shop, preparing it for the hours and hours of labor the harvesting would require.

The Claas Harvester with its eight-row corn header was greased and inspected from one end to the other, hoping to make it through its rigorous task without any major breakdowns. Trucks to haul the loads from the fields to the silage pit were worked on, along with the large John Deere tractor that would pack down the shredded corn as it was dumped into the pit, creating a huge mound of feed for the hungry cows. Extra truck drivers were hired to keep the chopper constantly going from morning to well after dark. It took an especially skilled operator to precisely cut the rows and rows of each field consisting of over 120 acres, making sure the truck was evenly spaced away from the chopper and the corn was fed evenly over into the bed of the truck as it loaded on-the-go.

Most of the time, Jim had run the chopper himself, putting in all the grueling hours nonstop, only pausing for a few minutes a day to cram down a sandwich I would bring to the field or to drink water from a jug packed with ice at the beginning of each day. This job was extremely tasking on a fully-healthy, strapping young man.

I glanced over at my husband and sized up the situation in my mind. Jim was sixty years old, had just endured three months of proton radiation treatments, and had a cancerous tumor in his brain. His eyesight was beginning to change, and I noticed very small differences in his memory function. How could he possibly be up to such a daunting task? But as I looked again at this man who did not even know the meaning of the word quit, I knew one thing for sure. He was going to go back to the job which defined exactly who he was, and he would give it his all. And there was nothing I could or would do to stop him.

We were returning to the farm and entering into THE HARVEST OF HOPE. Hope for our very uncertain future. Hope he would be given the supernatural strength and endurance to accomplish this great task just one more time. Because despite the grinding hours and challenges which loomed before us, my husband needed to accomplish this more than anything he had ever done before in his life.

Over eight hours later, I slid the key into the front door of our home we had left behind quite hastily a few months before. Jim was exhausted from the long drive but had insisted we travel straight through. It seemed so quiet and empty, as our son had taken our lab and St. Bernard dogs home with him to Texas when he had left a few weeks before. I couldn't wait to crawl into our own bed for a few hours of exhausted sleep after driving all that distance.

Switching on the entry-way light, I suddenly stopped dead in my tracks and gasped in horror! Every surface of my clean, orderly house was covered with dead flies! The furniture, the carpets, the cabinets, the table. We regularly had a pesticide service spray our house, as we lived only a short distance from the huge dairy barn and right in front of a field of alfalfa. Bugs, especially flies, were a natural part of our existence on a dairy farm. But NOT in my house. And NOT NOW!

Although our house was fairly new and there had not been a single window left open, somehow there had been an inlet for a few of those pesky insects to enter. Over a few days, they must have populated, then died rapidly from the pest control substance.

It really didn't matter how it had happened, the reality was I had to deal with it, and quickly. My husband needed a clean, restful place to sleep, and so did I.

For a brief moment, I teetered between utter hysteria and control. In the end, control won out, and I set about the tedious task of vacuuming and cleaning every room in my house. I started in the bedroom and attacked the master bathroom, stripping the bed and wiping down every surface with disinfectant cleaner so my husband could get into bed and rest. Once I had him safely tucked in, I closed the bedroom door, threw up a desperate prayer for the strength to finish this seemingly unending task before me, and put on my Walkman earphones. I cranked up the volume, listening to the most upbeat music I could find. I kept repeating to myself a Bible verse which seemed to fit this ridiculous occasion: "The joy of the Lord is my strength."

Several hours later, I crawled into bed, satisfied I had sanitized the entire house. Minutes before falling into a deep, deep sleep of exhaustion, I remember smiling tersely to myself and wondering if this awful, unexpected homecoming was a sign of many challenging things to come.

Chapter 20
The Last Harvest

October, 2010

HELP CAN ARRIVE IN A TIME of need from many sources. That corn harvest produced not only a bumper crop of feed but also an abundance of extraordinary generosity from some remarkably special people in our lives. My sis and brother-in-law traveled down from Kansas to pitch in. Charlie helped out in the fields and drove into town to pick up needed parts for the unexpected breakdowns. Lin helped in the scale house weighing the trucks, preparing and delivering food to our hungry men, and doing whatever needed to be done to keep our household running. They both provided much-needed moral support and love during the long days and nights.

My badminton partner and friend, Jerry, who had never stepped foot on a farm before, called to offer any help we could use. He proved to be invaluable in the scale house, relieving my sister for a few hours, collecting samples from the trucks to be tested in the microwave inside the scale house for moisture content, making sure the corn was neither too wet or too dry for the silage pit, weighing trucks, and inspiring us all with his positive spirit. The owner of the dairy and farm came out to the field and relieved Jim on the chopper many hours to give him a much-needed break.

Our regular employees tackled their jobs with loyalty, skill, persistence, and great camaraderie. Most of them had worked with us for years, and we weren't just employer/employees, we were personal friends. They had sorely missed their boss over the last few months, and we respected and cared for each one of them. We all became driven in this mission of bringing in this harvest together.

Halfway through the corn cutting, a few of the alfalfa fields had grown tall enough to cut one last time before going into their winter dormancy. This meant that my primary job on the farm of cutting the hay took precedence over my time for the remainder of the harvest. Realizing this would probably be the last time I would cut these fields brought an overwhelming sadness to my heart. One day, after receiving a timely email about hope from a friend, this was my reply:

I just opened and read the article on HOPE that you sent, and it was just what I needed to hear today.

I spent the whole day yesterday wiping these pesky drops from my eyes that kept blurring my vision of the field I was cutting. I have really not let it out for months for more than a couple of minutes at a time, when I could go into the bathroom and quickly cover it up so Jim would see only optimism and encouragement and strength from me. But yesterday, there was just no stopping it. A steady leakage like a dripping, annoying faucet.

That's what happens when a person gets too tired to hold it back!

I loved the great reminder to set goals, no matter what the situation.

In short, it truly did give me HOPE again!

The rain is falling down. I may get a day or so of rest.

Thanks again.

Blessings to You, Barb

After finishing the corn, our workers would switch over to the task of raking, baling, and hauling in the hay to stack inside the sheds. Getting this cutting of hay accomplished marked the conclusion to another long season of production from this sandy, parched land. This old soil was brought to life and fertility by water, nutrients, seed, and the mighty toil and sweat of many workers. I am proud to say my husband left a huge part of himself on this ancient land—a pathway used by Pueblo Indians making their way to the salt lakes located a few miles east of this area. Each acre had a story, and, over the course of ten years, we became a part of this land's saga.

Sheer determination had carried my husband through the long days of harvest, and finally the last bale of alfalfa was in the shed. The huge sheets of white plastic were spread over the gigantic pit of ensilage, held down by hundreds of old used tires retained on the farm for this purpose. Although every single person who had participated in this great accomplishment was tired to the bone, Jim was beyond fatigued. We had continued the juice routine and supplements for extra nourishment, but another regimen of the oral chemo pills began to take their effect on his already-ravaged, exhausted body.

There had been a couple of noticeable incidents during the harvest time which suggested the tumor had slightly affected him both physically and mentally. He had always been adept at math. Now, he struggled to figure out a chemical formula which would have previously been easy for him.

One Sunday afternoon, the man who could operate and repair every single machine on the place, ran one of the small swathers into the garage door on the side of the shop building. I could tell his reflexes weren't responding normally. But overall, he had accomplished the big goal, and there was huge satisfaction within his soul. We would just have to wait and see what happened in the coming days.

The next few weeks began to tell the story. At first, I was totally thankful to see Jim come home for a short nap in the middle of the afternoon or stay a little longer after lunch for a period of rest before driving the short distance back to the shop. Finally, he was following the doctor's advice about taking the time he needed to let his body regenerate and recover.

By this time, I had thoroughly educated myself on the chemo portion of his treatment, and I was more than a little concerned. I knew in many types of cancer, it was instrumental in bringing about remission. But, I also read much material about the extremely controversial side of the drug, and the massive side effects involved with its use.

Every single situation is unique and individual, and I began to weigh out both the positives and the negatives when it came down to my husband. I kept returning to the main goal we had set for his journey with cancer. This was the quality of life. After completing the full second round of oral chemo, I began to see the poisonous effects of chemo taking its toll on his body. It obviously was a direct side effect from the chemo and not the regrowth of the tumor. The proton radiation had significantly shrunk the original size of the tumor, and it had not had time to grow back this quickly.

Over the course of the next few weeks, I witnessed increasing fatigue and weakness. By this time, he could only muster enough energy to go up to the shop in the mornings. Yet another round of chemo was to begin soon. Would his body be able to handle it and continue to function well enough to do his job?

Our first big decision became clear to us when Jim came down with bronchitis the first week in November. Our local doctor loaded him up with antibiotics to get him over it as quickly as possible. Although my big strong husband tried to valiantly fight through it, his weakened body was very slow to respond. He was pale and listless. His cough became deep and relentless. He had to stay in bed most of the hours of the day. One of the worst side effects of chemo is the compromise to the immune system, making a person highly susceptible to any and all bad germs going around.

We sat on the couch one night and discussed the situation thoroughly. We listed the pros and cons, all that I had read, and every piece of advice given by friends and family on the subject. We weighed the advice of the physicians. Most of all, we discussed what we felt was best for us. Once the decision was made to stop the chemo, we never looked back. We felt a tremendous peace wash over us, and knew it was what we were supposed to do.

The second decision was excruciating for Jim. The very thought of giving up this life occupation, which was as much a part of him as breathing, tore through his heart and left an indelible scar. It came down to an ethical dilemma core to his character. Should he continue to take a large salary for a significant position he could no longer function at with one hundred percent capability? Other less ethical men would have hung on longer. He could not inflict this diminished production situation on his generous employer, who had bent over backward to accommodate and reward him. Again, a big discussion occurred between us.

"How soon should we leave? Where will we go?" The pained expression on his face told the story.

Of course, we had known this was a strong possibility. This wasn't a huge surprise, but it had seemed to happen much more quickly than we had considered it would. Our concentration had been so focused on achieving the completion of the harvest, the reality of physically moving from our home of over ten years, when it became right down to it, was a considerable shock to both of us. My mind had been exploring all the possibilities, but those possibilities were now a naked, raw reality.

Once again, the direction came clear to us. One day, during a phone call with our oldest son, he offered for us to come and live with him for a while. His beautiful, spacious, two-story home was located in the countryside near a town in eastern Kansas. He was going through a difficult divorce and I could hear the sincerity in his voice:

"You can stay in my basement in the spare bedroom with the bath and we can store all your furniture and boxes in my big shed. The kids will be there on most weekends, and I know they would love for you guys to come. Mom, you can even cook for us." The last part was said with a smile, knowing that cooking was neither my favorite or best attribute.

Once the big decision was made, I had to shift into another gear. It seemed like I had been doing that too many times in the last few months. I again realized we were on a bizarrely new, unknown path with every turn bringing extreme circumstances of change. I suddenly realized we would soon be having to say goodbye to many people we had come to dearly love.

Being so far away from family, we had developed close relationships with many people both on and off the farm: our workers, our Bible study group, my badminton friends, and Jim's fellow local farmers and neighbors. They were all special, wonderful individuals, living in a small-town atmosphere, and we had gone through so much together. As the word quickly spread throughout the community that we were moving, all those people rallied around us. In the next couple of weeks, many of them came to help us pack. They brought out meals to our house, and my friend Nancy planned a big going-away party in our honor.

Our employer told us while we were away, he and his wife had decided to sell the dairy and farm at the end of the year, factoring in the strong possibility we would probably have to be leaving soon anyway. They had already talked about retiring earlier, but our situation gave them added incentive to proceed with that plan. It gave Jim a sense of relief to know he would not be leaving them in a bind, trying to quickly replace him. Again, their extreme generosity came through as they assured us we would be paid our full salary through the end of the year, a whole month longer than we would even be there!

In our sorrow, we were lifted up once again by the blessings of good people and a merciful Lord, providing exactly what we needed and beyond.

Chapter 21
The Sad Good-bye

November, 2010

LIFE HAD TAKEN ON A HECTIC pace now that the big decision to leave New Mexico was finalized. Two of our three sons would be arriving soon from Kansas and Texas to complete the packing and load up our belongings. They were best able to take some time off from their jobs around the Thanksgiving holiday, so we chose to depart the day after Thanksgiving. Our wonderful daughter-in-law and two granddaughters were also coming to help. When I mentioned the actual date we planned to depart to my best friend Dorothy, she immediately came up with the sweetest gift anyone could have given us during this stressful time.

"Since your house is going to be all packed up, I want you and your family to come eat Thanksgiving dinner with us. I'm already cooking a big meal for part of our family. So please come and join us before you leave."

I had been so busy trying to figure out how we would achieve the daunting task of packing, the thought of a Thanksgiving meal had not even occurred to me. Dorothy's gift of hospitality was not only demonstrated by her delicious New Mexico culinary skills, but her gracious manner and hospitality was beyond compare. How blessed I felt to be fortunate enough to know her as my special forever friend. I couldn't imagine a better way to end our time in this extraordinary 'Land of Enchantment.'

Jim had only begun to recover from the first round of bronchitis a couple of days before our farewell party. Up until the last few hours before it was time to go, he planned to push his way through it. After all, he was one of the honored guests, and it would probably be the last time he might see most of these wonderful friends. But as the time drew closer for our departure, I could sense that even our 'superman' could not muster the energy to do this. Our son Chad offered to stay home with him while Shana and the girls would go with me. I started to get a sick feeling in the pit of my stomach, an uneasiness I couldn't shake.

The party can only be described with adjectives such as sad, memorable, poignant. From early evening until almost 8:30 p.m., the food and fellowship flowed with sweet communion. I couldn't believe the number of people whose lives had touched ours during our ten years in this beautiful state--from my badminton friends who I had sweated, played, and laughed with three days a week for hours on end, to members of the historical Coronado Women's Club which I had joined several years back, and to our loving Bible study friends we had worshipped and shared intimate prayer requests with for many years.

They all came with their best wishes and love. From natives whom had lived in the area all their lives to recent replants from all over the United States coming to find peace and contentment in a retirement development, this small community was both diverse and unique. But the common thread of acceptance and friendship had certainly been extended to Jim and me. Many of Jim's personal farmer friends were disappointed he had been unable to come, but Shana took pictures of every guest with me so he could see how many people came to show us love and support.

As I later looked at every picture, I saw both smiles and tears, summing up the mood of the night. Our special friend Zona, who had just gone through extensive chemo treatment battling her own war with non-Hodgkin's lymphoma, arrived with a turban on her head to cover her cute little bald head. She had become like another mom to both of us over the years. Shortly after we became friends, she lost her precious Phillip, and from that time on, we were always there for each other. We took care of her, and she took care of us as true family did. The thought of leaving her behind, especially in her condition, broke our hearts.

Shortly after we left, she flew to Washington to live out the remainder of her days with her son and family. When the night finally drew to an end, I was emotionally exhausted, but also completely bowled over by the support I had received that evening. I only wished my husband could have drawn in all the love and encouragement to help carry him through the most difficult days ahead.

My boys and family were tireless as they packed, wrapped, boxed, and loaded the entire contents of our home, storage shed, Jim's office, and outdoor items into the trailers and pickup beds. Our plan was to caravan out of New Mexico shortly after partaking of Dorothy's delicious meal on Thanksgiving Day. Jim and I would take our time, driving the SUV and stopping for frequent breaks. The others, along with one of our farmer friends who had volunteered to drive his pickup and trailer, would deadhead it to Kansas, only stopping for minimum breaks.

Instead of regaining his strength from the first bout with bronchitis, the symptoms came back with a vengeance. The chemo pills had left Jim's body unable to defend itself against the attack. He became much worse quite suddenly, and our primary care physician recommended we take him into the ER in Albuquerque to treat the illness with IV meds. What awful timing, as it was the day before Thanksgiving, and all our plans were shot through. Of course, the only important priority was restoring my husband's health back to a condition where he could make the long ride up to Kansas.

As we had found out before, there is certain criteria to be met before a person can be admitted to the hospital. After waiting a few hours back in an ER receiving room, we were told Jim's fever was one point less than what is required for admittance. Therefore, the ER doctor would treat him with IV antibiotics in our tiny cubicle for several hours, run him through a course of blood tests, and then reevaluate his condition.

My head swam with dread as I stared at the tiny straight-back chair sitting beside the hospital bed and heard the screams for help in the curtained cubicle next to ours. Already beyond fatigue myself from the days of packing, I could only numbly sit in the hard chair and lean my head on the side of Jim's bed. Tears of frustration began to course down my cheeks. I certainly didn't want to go out to the ER waiting room where a couple dozen accident-related and sick cases were sitting. All I could do was endure and hang on for the next few hours.

The yelling and screaming in the next cubicle over continued relentlessly, and through the flimsy curtain I could hear the nurse telling the irate woman they would not be giving her the drugs she pled for. I concluded this woman must be a 'regular' at the ER, coming in when she no longer could obtain her drugs on the street. As the hours passed by, I overheard several other conversations coming from the various cubicles. All kinds of circumstances which probably occurred routinely every single night in the busy ER area of a big city.

By now, my head was beginning to throb and my scratchy throat began to hurt. I felt low, sick, helpless, and isolated in the midst of the chaos all around me. I watched the monotonous drip of the IV as it slowly emptied the clear bag of liquid into my husband's vein and prayed for it to heal his body.

When morning finally came, and I felt it wasn't too early to call back home, I relayed the progress from the hospital, and we talked over Plan B. Obviously, Jim would not feel like either eating a big Thanksgiving meal or getting in a vehicle and traveling the many long hours to Kansas. But with everything packed up at the house, returning there was also not an option. And, with the hospital not admitting him into a regular room for recovery, the only alternative plan I could come up with was to rent a motel room for us there in Albuquerque where he could rest until he felt well enough to travel.

Because my sons were on a tight schedule with their limited days off from their jobs, they agreed to go out to Dorothy's house to eat and then depart quickly on their journey northward.

I asked the Lord to help me find a nice available motel room on such short notice on the holiday—one with a huge king bed and no noisy neighbors. Once again, the provision was made smoothly and quickly, as I found a nice, quiet motel on the east side of Albuquerque in an area away from the busy interstate.

Once we were checked in and had eaten the food picked up at a drive-through restaurant, we both collapsed on the bed from sheer exhaustion. I was still extremely concerned about my husband's condition, praying the IV would be enough to turn him around. I knew by this time I was also coming down with something and asked the Lord to restore my health enough to get us through the long trip ahead—whenever we would feel well enough to depart. For now, I knew the best plan was to stay close to the hospital in case we needed to go back, concentrate on resting our exhausted bodies, and to lean hard into the Lord.

Waking up in a strange place a few hours later, it took several minutes to get my wits about me. Doubts and worries swirled in my brain, and the reality of our situation came crashing down all around me. We had been ripped from our place of security from every direction. We no longer had a job. We no longer had a home. We had said goodbye to our friends and neighbors, and our children were gone away from us. We had not been able to spend our last day in fellowship with our dearest friends. We had spent tortuous hours in a cold, crazy hospital ER cubicle. We were stuck in a motel room in a city for an undetermined amount of days. We were exhausted, sick, and isolated. It was almost more than I could bear!

It was one of the most difficult days we spent since this whole crazy ordeal had suddenly, without warning, been thrust upon us! That evening, for a long time, my husband and I let down and grieved together over the great loss of all we had known before. And the looming uncertainty of what the future held for us.

Two days passed before we both felt well enough to begin our journey up to our son's home. During those two days, Jim had taken the oral medications he had been prescribed upon being dismissed from the hospital, and I had loaded up on over-the-counter meds to deal with my symptoms.

We heard with great relief that the moving trucks and trailers had all arrived safely at Chris's home, the trailers were all unloaded into either the big shop or the house, and our bedroom would be organized and waiting for us upon our arrival. Our farmer friend had quickly unloaded his trailer and turned right around and driven straight back to New Mexico already.

I felt so blessed to know we had raised such great sons willing to take care of us in our dire time of need. They, along with our daughter-in-law, had done above and beyond all we needed them to do in the last few days. We could not have accomplished this move without them. I thanked God for their strong work ethic, and the ability to accomplish a big task—both attributes they had seen their dad live out before them all their lives.

Before leaving New Mexico, we had taken one last quick drive through the farm. Once again, tears welled up as the realization fully hit us both that this chapter of our lives was forever closed. The house looked cold and empty. There was a brisk, cold wind blowing out of the north. The fields lay barren from the final, completed harvest. We wouldn't be around to watch them change again, creating the brand-new season of renewal and growth, awakening the stunned dormant alfalfa and turning it green and fragrant with ladybugs and butterflies dancing all around in the warm spring breezes.

We wouldn't be there to see the small herds of antelope nibbling on the fresh growth, or watch the ravens take a ride atop the irrigation towers as they slowly circled the fields of short shoots of corn, bursting through the soil in evenly-spaced rows. We wouldn't be witnessing the striking, gorgeous, New Mexico sunsets which took our breath away. Behind us lay the familiarity of a lifestyle we had lived for almost forty years. We drove out of the farm into a foreign land of precarious uncertainty.

Chapter 22
The Love of Family

IT TOOK US TWO WHOLE DAYS to reach our son's home. I had driven about half-way there the first day until we both felt we could go no further without rest. We were both still recovering from our illnesses, and Jim remained extremely weak and tired. The further north we traveled, the colder the temperature became.

Finally pulling into the driveway of the place we would call home for the next few months, we were greeted with a large welcoming party of family. The shouts and sweet kisses of the grandkids, the warm hugs of our children, and the fragrant aroma of food created a soft buffer to the harsh reality of our loss.

As they proudly led us down the stairs to our bedroom, we marveled at the way they had paid such extraordinary attention to detail to make it truly feel like home. Our own bedroom set was neatly arranged down to our own bedding and snugly quilt. A few of our personal decorating items and lamps were placed upon the dresser and night stands, and even one of our favorite paintings had been hung on the wall.

How they had found all these items amongst the hundreds of boxes was amazing in itself! Supper was ready and waiting for us upstairs in the kitchen. Although the children had already been fed, the food had been kept warm on the stove for us. I could not thank them enough for all they done in the past couple of weeks. As I lay in my bed under clean warm covers, I again thanked God for the precious gift of my loving family, and drifted into an exhausted sleep of warm, welcome peace.

The positive aspect of this move was that we did not have to unpack anything other than our winter clothes and personal items. It was a good thing, as it took several days just to recover from the hospital, the moving process, and the physical and emotional trauma of sickness and loss. We soon fell into a daily routine. Chris arose early each morning, showered, and left for work. Jim and I had a leisurely morning, sometimes sleeping in late in the quiet house, sometimes getting up and eating a home-cooked breakfast or brunch.

After climbing the basement stairs, I soon took on the morning routine of cleaning and stoking the large wood fireplace. As soon as the fire was burning hot enough, the fan would kick on and circulate the warm air throughout the house through the vent system, quickly taking off the chill. The cold weather settled into those Kansas plains with a vengeance that winter bringing an extra amount of snow with it. Retrieving logs from the stack outside, building a new fire when it burned out, and keeping the fire burning well throughout the day was almost a full-time job it seemed, but I didn't mind the work at all. I missed all the activities, work, and exercise with my friends.

Besides my son and family, we knew no one in this midwestern town. Our days were filled with long, quiet hours. Late in the afternoon, I would begin preparing an evening meal for the three of us, and after supper we would relax in the living room, either watching TV or reading. When Jim's body became strong enough, we would take a walk to the end of the long driveway up to the mailbox at the road and back or walk across the back field of our son's home if the weather allowed.

Sometimes, Jim would amble down to the shop, poking around in our boxes looking for a particular item, or just sitting in his farm pickup. More than once, I would realize he had been outside for too long in the cold and go out looking to make sure he was all right. A couple of times I found him sound asleep, sitting in the driver's seat with his head leaning forward on the steering wheel. Once when this happened, I opened the door and felt his cold hands and face. It was concerning to me, but I knew he just wanted to sit in the familiar seat which mentally took him back to the farm he so dearly missed.

With his eyesight gradually getting worse and his reaction time diminishing, we had made an agreement that I would do all the driving from now on. Just to make sure he remembered, Chris and I had found an out-of-the-way place to keep his keys. I slowly began to realize how the dynamics between us were changing. I had to think more about what was logical and safe for his well-being and make more of the decisions about our changing lives.

In looking at the days ahead, one of my desires was to take Jim on a once-in-a-lifetime trip he would particularly enjoy. I wanted to fulfill one of the items on his bucket list. In years past, we had tossed around the idea of someday retiring, buying a big camper, and traveling across the country like so many other retirees. There were still many parts of this great land we had never seen, and loving the outdoors as we both did, it seemed like a perfect fit for us. Would it still be a possibility now to fulfill this dream, if only for a little while?

One day, as we discussed this very subject, I could see Jim's eyes begin to light up. I had thrown out a few possibilities including a cruise, or a big trip by airplane to a beautiful resort somewhere. But the travel trailer pushed a button within Jim's mind, and in the days ahead, it became an obsession. He spent hours on the computer, looking at all the types and styles and prices. When he read about an RV show coming up soon in Wichita, he got very excited about going. He also wanted to go to the RV sales places in the area, to personally see what was available.

At first, I thought it could be a good possibility. I knew I would have to do the driving, but with my experience with driving large farm machines, the idea did not intimidate me. As we seriously began to pursue the idea, doubts began to creep in. Campers and RVs had become big ticket items, as we discovered in our exploration on the internet. They also had many complicated features which required some physical strength and agility, like leveling, setting up, and dumping refuse.

It would also be beneficial to have a good co-pilot to direct and help with the backing and parking into RV spaces. And what if we were out on the road and Jim became quite ill? We might need medical care located far from a remote campsite. And in a practical sense, what would I do with the camper in the future? It was a big investment I might not be able to get back. After thinking more carefully and discussing this with my boys, I realized it would not be the wise decision to make.

When I broke the news to Jim and told him I thought we should explore a single trip instead, he immediately became furious! Did I know how much time he had spent searching and looking for this? If I wasn't all for it, why had I let him pursue the idea and get his hopes up? Although I carefully tried to explain my reasoning without hurting his pride, he refused to see the logic. He truly felt like he could easily handle it all, including the backing and the leveling and all the other aspects. And why would I think he might need sudden medical care? He would be perfectly fine. He sat in his chair and sulked for hours and days.

It was a hard lesson for me to come to terms with. In a way, he was right. I had allowed him to dream an unrealistic dream. But I was new to this shift of responsibility and was learning along the way how hard it was to have to be the one to make the hard choices. Even though I knew it was for the best, I hated seeing the disappointed countenance on his face. At this point, I would have given him the moon if I could have done it. But in the long run, I knew the right decision had been made.

I waited a while before I brought up the subject of a trip again. I knew he would not be open to anything I suggested until he got over his disappointment. In the meantime, Christmas had stolen upon us, and I wanted it to be the most special one ever. Family, food, decorations, games, and laughter. We all needed a big dose of celebration together, especially after the Thanksgiving disaster.

It ended up being a series of events, including our extended families on both sides of the family. Although our Texas son and family had taken off extensive time to help us move, a very understanding boss allowed them more time to come back during the Christmas break. We treasured every single moment together. What would 365 days bring about? Would we all be together again this time next year? I tried not to think about it, instead living in the present. But I couldn't stop the nagging thought from occasionally surfacing.

Jim had wanted to shop for my Christmas gift, but we were afraid for him to venture out into the crowds. There was too big of a risk he could pick up some more of those dangerous germs. In fact, we had rarely been out in public since our arrival in Kansas. We missed attending church and being around people in general.

Several weeks before Christmas, he had begun to see frequent commercials with pretty models in snuggly warm pink footie pajamas. Knowing how cold-natured I was, particularly during this extra cold winter in Kansas, he decided it would be the perfect present. But when he tried to order it with the number on the screen, he had difficulty with the credit card and ordering process. One day he came to me and shared his frustration with me.

"I really wanted this to be a surprise, but I'm gonna need your help with the order. For some reason, I can't seem to get the numbers right."

"It's fine, honey. It's the thought that counts, and you couldn't have come up with a more perfect idea. The basement bedroom is cold, and this will keep me so warm and snugly!"

I began to realize both his eyesight and his ability to read factual information was beginning to be affected. I began to think of ways I could bring peace and comfort to his frustration. I had noticed that although he still tried to read the local newspaper, he picked it up less and less. Watching TV and napping had begun to take up much of his time.

During the long cold, wintry evenings, I began reading him a book out loud entitled *90 Minutes in Heaven: A True Story of Death and Life* by Don Piper. It was a story about a man involved in a horrific car crash who had been pronounced dead, only to come back to life an hour and a half later, claiming to have seen Heaven. It was a beautiful story of faith and hope, with a detailed description of what awaited my husband on the other side. It took us many nights of reading to finish the book. As I read, I could feel Jim's attitude relax, and many times I saw him close his eyes as he peacefully listened. Without a doubt, he wasn't the only one who benefited from those quiet nights of reading. I also began reading Scripture, especially focusing on the powerful promises found in Psalms.

After the holidays, we finally began to discuss special trips again. We wanted to include family in one, and then do a big trip with just the two of us. As we had experienced a cruise years earlier with many of our New Mexico friends, it seemed like this might be just the ticket. Staying in one room for the entire time was certainly appealing, and we would have the choice of doing as little or as much as we wanted. This flexibility would allow for days when all Jim might feel like doing would be walking across the ship to a restaurant or sitting in a lounge chair soaking up the warm sun.

As we studied all the different destinations on the computer, he finally chose the two-week cruise which left Florida, went through the

Panama Canal, and ended up in Los Angeles, where we would catch a flight home to Kansas City. After talking to our cruise consultant, I was assured this would be a feasible trip for us to take. I talked over our situation with her, explaining that at times we might even need a wheelchair if we had to go long distances from the ship to the airport, etc.

She also gave me great confidence that in the case of any medical emergency, not only was there medical help onboard, but also the capability to fly us off the ship. We booked the trip on faith, dearly hoping that between this time and April, Jim's condition would hold up.

Chapter 23
The Great Reveal

Spring, 2011

FEBRUARY BROUGHT AROUND our forty-first wedding anniversary on Valentine's Day. As winter slowly transitioned into springtime, we began walking every day in the afternoons when the temperature was highest. Slow strolls up to the mailbox, then circling back down to the house or out to the back field. The fresh air and sunshine felt wonderful for both body and soul. Sometimes we walked in peaceful silence and other times we shared our thoughts and feelings.

One bright day in March, with the soft southern breeze blowing as we slowly meandered up the driveway, I began to open up about some very private thoughts I had been experiencing relating to all we were going through.

"I guess one of the most difficult parts of this whole big journey is the unknown. Wouldn't it be good if we could just see into the future and definitely know what our timeline is so we could know exactly where to go from this point? How long we should plan on staying here with Chris . . . whether we should plan on trying to find a house somewhere to live in . . . just knowing what to do in general. I just wish God would tell us specifically how much time we have . . . ."

Suddenly Jim stopped and looked directly into my eyes. "What if I told you that I pretty well know the answers to your questions?"

I started to dismiss his remark, but suddenly I felt a jolt go through me.

"What do you mean, you know the answers?" I asked, staring hard at him.

"I mean, I pretty well know what's going to happen."

I bowed my head, and thought to myself, *Yes, we both know the sad outcome of this horrible circumstance we are in.*

But when I looked up again, I saw Jim was struggling internally, and suddenly I knew he was trying to think of just the right words to use.

"What if I told you that God directly spoke to me and told me what was going to happen?"

I grabbed hold of both of his hands and looked deeply into his troubled eyes.

"Tell me exactly what you're talking about! What do you mean, God spoke to you directly? And when did this happen?"

"It happened when you were in Kansas and I was back home in New Mexico by myself. One night, I got woke up by a voice inside my head. At first, I thought I was dreaming, but I wasn't. I was told that I had less than two years to live, and I needed to love my family more than I ever had before. That was pretty much all that was said." He looked down and began to start to walk again.

"Whoa, wait a minute! You're telling me you knew this was going to happen several months before you were even diagnosed with cancer? And, Jim, why in the world haven't you told me about this before?"

He stopped again and shook his head.

"I've thought about it so many times and started to tell you. At first, I began to doubt it even really happened, but then when I got this tumor, I knew that it was real. I can't really explain it, but I guess the main reason I didn't tell you was that I thought if you knew about it, you might just tell me to accept it. That it was just God's will for me to die. That you wouldn't fight as hard for me, trying every way we could to cure this. I don't want to die yet! I want to watch my grandkids grow up!"

Tears welled up in his eyes, and my heart broke in two at that moment. Tears started streaming down my face, but suddenly something huge occurred to me.

"You should know I would not ever tell you to just lay down and die. You should know me well enough to know that I would explore every avenue to fight this thing. But I need for you to look at this another way. God did not HAVE to reveal this to you. Don't you see, the God of the Universe cared enough about you to actually take the time to SPEAK to YOU!

"If this doesn't prove not only that He is real, but also He loved you enough to do this, I don't know what will. The question is, WHY did he choose to do it? As I'm standing here, I think I know at least part of the answer. I remember when I came back home with you after Christmas last year and I got sick with the mono. I saw a BIG change in you as you responded to the whole situation. You took care of me with a tenderness and love I had never seen in you before.

"It helps to prove your encounter WAS real. Those were some of the best times of our marriage. I saw a new sweetness, a new attitude in you. I even told one of my friends how wonderful and close the last few months had been for us. And secondly, it occurs to me you should tell your children about this. It could increase their faith, instead of letting this experience turn them bitter and angry. It would glorify God and show how personal and loving and real He is!"

I shook my head in wonder over and over again as we finished our walk. I could scarcely take it all in. God had spoken to my husband. This was not something he would make up, and I had witnessed the great change in him personally. How many people on this earth were so privileged to know the future?

Of course, immediately I began to calculate the time in my head. He had gotten the message in late November of 2010. A year and full three months had already passed by, meaning we had less than nine months remaining, and it could be less than that. The reality hit me hard. We wouldn't be having another Christmas all together. In a few months, I would be living a completely different life alone for the first time in over forty years. Only with the Lord's help could I endure what lay ahead. But, looking behind, I saw how His great provision had carried us through so far. I had to trust like never before.

Many tears and thoughts streamed from my heart and mind all evening. Before we went to sleep that night, once again, I assured my husband I would be there for him in every way I possibly could. Again, we talked about sharing this experience with each one of the boys. Jim finally understood how important it was for each one of them to hear this directly from his personal account. They knew their dad and his character of honesty. Hearing this from his own lips would be so much more effective than me telling them about it much later.

Our faith in the Lord was the most important quality we could pass down to our children and grandchildren. Somehow, this whole tragic experience began to take on a semblance of purpose and direction, even if we might never have all the answers to our questions.

Within the next couple of weeks, Jim intentionally shared this very personal experience with each one of our children. We left it up to the Lord to speak to their hearts individually. We knew our part was to share this revelation with them, but they each had to decide what to do with it. We trusted this testimony of faith would be passed down through the generations to come as a great legacy of their Papa Jim's life and strong belief in God.

Toward the end of March, we drove down to Texas and had a family time of enjoyment at the Great Wolf Lodge in Grapevine. We all stayed in the lodge and ate and played together in the adjoining indoor waterpark. It was a memorable time with grandchildren, kids, and grandparents all having joyful fun together. For a few days, we almost forgot about the cancer. From bedtime stories with woodsy puppets in pajamas to careening down twisting slides of water, we put aside the heaviness of this great valley of life we were all experiencing. It was just what we all needed.

The only time reality came into focus was one brief incident when Jim left the waterpark to go to the men's room and was gone too long. One of the boys found him wandering through the hallways trying to find his way back to the waterpark area. It was a solemn reminder the tumor was probably beginning to grow back and cloud his sense of direction. I thought ahead to our big cruise coming up in less than a month and prayed it would all be possible.

For six months and holding, Jim's quality of life had remained pretty good, and we were extremely pleased. That had been the ultimate goal of going the route of proton radiation. With no regrets of the choices we had made, we knew the most difficult days were coming soon.

The weeks went by quickly as we prepared for our big trip. The big house our son graciously shared with us was quiet and private during the week, but loud and boisterous on the weekends when his children came to stay with him. We cherished the times when we could watch the grandchildren playing and laughing and sitting together around the dining room table with us. From that table we all played some of our favorite board games, we formed play dough into all kinds of animals and shapes, and we watched our youngest granddaughter and grandson blow out the candles on their birthday cakes that spring.

I noticed Jim began having a little trouble with all the noise of a house full of children, but he wasn't about to complain. Sometimes he would retreat to his recliner or go down to the bedroom to rest. His nerves seemed to be a little on edge, and he began to have an annoying headache at times. But those grandchildren were his life and joy. I started to realize the time was coming, maybe after the trip, that we might need to make an adjustment in our living arrangements. My sister and I began to talk about us moving to the town she lived in, which was also where my mom and some of our other relatives lived. I began to envision another change coming to our lives.

Chapter 24
The Cruise into Transition

April, 2011

AT LAST THE BIG DAY ARRIVED for us to drive to the Kansas City airport for our flight to Florida to board the big cruise ship. Packing for a two-week vacation was no small feat, especially with the small pharmacy of medications and supplements we had to take along. I felt a little anxious as we took off on the long flight. It was going to be just Jim and me, and we were going to be a long, long ways from home and family. I just had to trust the Lord would be with us every hour of every day we were gone, and this would be a wonderful, memorable special time. A once-in-a-lifetime trip of relaxation and fun.

The flight was uneventful, and thankfully, we had found a connecting flight allowing us to stay on the same plane. The transport van which drove us to our hotel in Miami was easy to find upon arrival and, although we were exhausted, we were able to enjoy a nice dinner in the motel restaurant before collapsing on the bed in our room. As we didn't have to embark to the ship until late the next afternoon, we looked forward to a leisurely, morning stroll on the famous Miami Beach Boardwalk just behind our hotel. I was so happy our cruise consultant had been so efficient at setting up all the details of our trip.

It was a bright, sunny Florida day and we were excited to board the ocean cruiser. We had anticipated this trip for many cold, wintry Kansas days, and as the huge ship finally pulled away from Miami, we sat on the top deck and soaked up the warm sunshine as we leisurely watched the departure. Our bags would be arriving at our cabin door within the next couple of hours, and we began to feel ourselves slipping into the laid-back cruise mentality. The only schedule we were on was what our tummies dictated, and the hardest choices we had to make were which of the many enticing restaurants to indulge in.

Purposefully, we had chosen only a couple of excursions to participate in when the ship docked in various locations along the route. Factoring in the heat and fatigue, staying mostly on the air-conditioned ship with all the various array of activities and entertainment offered daily was the best choice for us. With twelve decks to explore and a huge theater area featuring various live entertainment shows each night, we wouldn't be bored, yet our little private room was available for a nap whenever needed.

Every morning, a daily schedule with hour-by-hour available activities was delivered to our room by the steward who constantly monitored our every need. Each time we arrived back at our room, a nice little surprise awaited us—from the chocolate strawberries which greeted us the first day to various animal- shaped towels placed on our freshly-made beds. We were properly spoiled!

For the first few days, our trip was all I had dreamed it would be. Other than the extra naps Jim's body required, it seemed like the trip would be seamless. Jim especially enjoyed indulging in the delicious food available. One night we celebrated our long-overdue wedding anniversary at the onboard steakhouse. We dressed up, had our picture taken by the photographer on the spiral staircase of the ship, and topped the night off with a special little anniversary cake our cruise consultant had arranged for us.

On day five, we spent the entire day being educated about and personally observing the interesting process of maneuvering our huge ship through the Panama Canal, considered one of the Seven Wonders of the Modern World. It was an incredible experience, and we were so happy we had chosen this cruise.

On day eight, the day after we had done a small excursion at the docking at Costa Rica, we walked to the middle of the ship to a small cafe for lunch. As we approached the check-in station to be seated, Jim suddenly tapped me on the shoulder and told me he needed to sit down . . . immediately!

I quickly led him to a small table and pulled out a chair for him. He leaned forward, placing his head in his hands. I told the waiter we would need to sit at this table and asked him to quickly bring us some glasses of water.

"Are you okay?" I asked him with concern.

"Just very light-headed and dizzy. Give me a minute."

When the waiter came to take our order, I told him we needed a few minutes as my husband was not feeling well. Jim had gone white as a sheet and was still holding his head.

"Do you need to go back to the room and lie down?"

"If I can make it there."

In my mind, I retraced our route to the end of the ship where we would enter the elevators which took us down several levels, and then our path through the narrow hallways to arrive at our room. The walk would normally take us about ten minutes, but suddenly it seemed like miles away.

"Well, let's sit here until you think you can make it. I can just order us some food to go."

As the minutes ticked by, my mind raced. What if Jim passed out? What if he couldn't walk all the way back to the room? Should I go find a wheelchair to take him back? By the time the food was done, his color was slowly returning, and he gave me a weak smile.

"Sorry I scared you. Are you ready to go?"

"Whenever you feel like it. Take as much time as you need. Do you think you can eat here, or shall we take it back to our room?"

"I'm better, but I think I still need to lie down for a while. Let's go."

We slowly walked back across the ship, stopping frequently to rest. Thankfully, there were benches placed along the main walkway. I was so relieved when we finally made it to our little private cabin. Jim fell asleep as soon as his head hit the pillow. I sat at the tiny desk in the only chair in the room and began to read the book I had brought along on the trip, but I couldn't concentrate very well. I just hoped this was an isolated incident brought on by fatigue from the excursion we had gone on the previous day.

The evening show on the ship that night was a circus act. We had gone every single night to the performances, which were each entertaining and varied. From a group impersonating the Beatles to a comedian to a hypnotist, we enjoyed them all. At the last minute when we were all dressed and ready to go, Jim told me to go on ahead and go by myself. He was feeling a little weak and tired. I protested, not wanting to leave him alone, but he insisted I go ahead, and he would stay in the room and rest.

Although I felt I should stay with him, he kept insisting I shouldn't have to spend more time cooped up in the small cabin, especially since I was all ready to go. Reluctantly I agreed and headed to the end of the ship by myself. Quarters were very close in the cabin, and it was nice to get out after spending several hours that afternoon just watching Jim sleep and trying to stay quiet and occupied.

As I arrived in the auditorium, the lights were already turned down, and the performance was just starting. The bottom floor of seating looked full, so I quickly got back into the elevator and went up a floor to the balcony area. After scanning the seats, I found an empty chair on the side and quietly slipped in. The circus act was fun to watch, and the two main performers were quite good and comical, too. I still felt uneasy about leaving Jim in the room the whole time I was at the show.

As soon as it was done, I hurriedly beelined it back to the room to check on him. When I knocked on the door, to my surprise, Jim was still dressed in the clothes he was going to wear to the show, and I sensed something was wrong. As I began to take off my shoes and get ready to change into something more comfortable, he asked me how I liked the show. I told him it was really good, and I was sorry he couldn't have enjoyed it with me.

"Well, I did see the show, and I saw you too!" He stated angrily.

I froze in place and looked intently at him.

"You mean you came to the show after all? If you saw me, why didn't you come sit beside me?" I asked.

"Yes, I saw you alright! And I saw you sitting up there in the front row, and I saw you watching that guy with the bright orange hair, and I saw you waiting for him after it was over!" He was visibly upset and angry.

But, to both of our surprise, I burst out laughing. What he had just said was so outlandish, I reacted before I could contain myself. The very picture of me having a 'thing' for the young man who was younger than my own boys with his spiked, bright -orange hair just suddenly struck me as hilarious.

"What are you talking about?" I exclaimed, still laughing. "I was sitting in the balcony, and I sure wasn't waiting for a circus performer after the show!"

"You're lying! I went to the show, and I sat back a few rows from you, and I saw you!" he exclaimed. "You always told me that when you were young, you wanted to be in the circus."

I burst out laughing again. This couldn't be happening!

"You really came to the show? Well, if you did, it wasn't me in the front row, and just the thought of me being attracted to a kid with bright orange hair is so totally ridiculous I can't even believe you would think such a thing. And, yes, when I saw an acrobatic trapeze act on TV when I was five, I really wanted to grow up and do that, but I was FIVE."

I looked at him and realized he wasn't believing a single thing I said, and suddenly it wasn't funny anymore. My mind was trying to figure out what was really happening to my husband and it began to sink in that for him to believe such an absurd concept was downright scary.

"Listen, Jim, I wasn't in the front row. I was in the balcony. I didn't go near the stage area, and right after the show I came down to our room as soon as I could get here. Your mind is playing tricks on you, and you have to understand that."

I got very close to his face and looked squarely into his eyes. I could see he was beginning to get a look of confusion on his face, and he became very quiet.

"Now if you want to keep discussing this, feel free to, but I've told you the truth and that's all there is to it. I'm sorry you got so upset. I believe this has happened because of the tumor. I truly hope you'll be able to understand that and get past it. We've got a few days left of this cruise, and I hope we can relax and enjoy it."

I felt him backing down, confused and conflicted, yet still wary and not totally convinced.

I went to bed that night with my own uneasiness and moments of sheer fear for what had occurred that evening. I was totally shaken. Was this going to continue throughout the remainder of the trip? Two certainties hit me. I was over 3000 miles away from Emporia, Kansas, and did not know a single soul on this huge cruise ship. I had to survive whatever came up the next five days until we got back on an airplane in Los Angeles, California, to fly back to Kansas City.

I only had one hope to cling to. God knew exactly the predicament I was in. He had been completely trustworthy throughout this long, impossible ordeal, and I had no reason to doubt He would come through once again. I prayed whatever pressure caused from the growth of Jim's brain tumor causing the illogical paranoia to take over his reasoning, would be stopped. I prayed I would be given strength to deal with each day, and wisdom to know exactly what to do. I asked God to provide me with the help I needed through people with compassionate hearts. And I promised myself and Him I wouldn't leave my husband alone again for a single minute the remainder of the cruise. As the gentle rocking of the ship lulled me into sleep at last, I felt the arms of my Savior comfort and sustain me.

Although Jim didn't bring up the strange events of the previous night, I could tell there remained some doubt in his mind. I determined to put the doubt to rest by being positive and upbeat about the remainder of our trip. We were to have a short docking in Guatemala on this day nine, and we decided to venture off the ship on foot for a short stroll through the various booths set up with homemade crafts by local artisans. We would not partake of the various excursions offered, but at least get off the ship for a break. Jim showed no signs of dizziness during our lunch at the huge cafeteria on the upper deck, and I thought the change in scenery might be good for both of us.

We picked up a few brightly-colored souvenirs; a doll for my mom's collection, a beautiful woven shoulder bag, and a small interesting painting depicting workers in a field. The locals were eager to show us their wares, but not smothering us with pressure to buy, and we enjoyed the experience. We got our picture taken with a small monkey dressed in a brightly colored shirt. We talked with one artist who spoke broken English and learned about his background and meager life in this very poor country.

After about an hour, Jim indicated his energy was diminishing quickly, so we slowly made our way back up the ramp into the ship. We headed for the cool refreshments on the open top deck and sat at a table with a big umbrella to shield us from the intense tropical heat.

Although my husband was very quiet most of the day, I determined to sweep away the remaining remnants of lingering paranoia he still exhibited through his facial expressions. I chatted about the only other excursion we had signed up for on our trip. On day eleven, we would arrive in Acapulco, Mexico, and go view the amazing, famous cliff divers. In our room, as Jim got ready for a nap, I pulled out the brochure and showed him the pictures of the divers sailing through the air from the steep perches on the narrow high cliffs. I told him I would check to see if we had to walk up any flights of stairs to view them, and if so, we could make arrangements for a wheelchair if he wasn't up to the climb. With disgust, he said he wouldn't need any help and wasn't about to be pushed in a wheelchair of all things! I told him there was no shame in getting assistance so he could enjoy the experience we had planned to see, but the anger started to show in his face again, so I dropped the subject.

I was already thinking ahead to the disembarkation at the end of our trip; about us standing in line with our carry-on bags; claiming our big bags in the luggage area; and the experience of walking a long distance through a huge unfamiliar airport. Somehow, I would have to convince Jim by that time he would need to get some help with this process. I would definitely need divine intervention to help me through that day!

As was the case in the last few months, I focused on taking life one day at a time. I sensed a new phase of our cancer experience had begun on day eight of our cruise. The doctors had explained that when the tumor began to grow back and push its way into different areas of the brain, changes would occur in both the physical and mental aspects. Depending on the area in which the tumor resided, each individual's experience would vary as to how they would be affected.

Jim's tumor lodged in the area of the brain that controlled vision, logic and reasoning, and motor control. Because of his recent behavior, I knew the tumor that had been shrunken in size by the proton radiation, was again resuming its growth. This was exactly what we had been told would happen. Of course, I had had no way of knowing when these changes in personality would show themselves. I had hoped we could make it through this last big trip together before we would have to start dealing with the changes which could radically change my husband's personality. It looked like we were about two weeks too late.

The reality of our situation hit me hard. I was full of questions I could not talk to anyone about until we arrived back in Kansas. The loneliness of my dilemma was unsettling and stressful. The realization that I had lost the person I had been married to for over forty years began to sink in. We were moving into the unpredictable unknown future. God help us!

The remainder of the trip was a confirmation of my suspicions. Although we were able to make it through the excursion of the cliff divers without the aid of a wheelchair, it was difficult and scary. We had climbed many steps, and with the necessary frequent stops to rest, we lagged behind the group. The big effort and expenditure of energy put a damper on the excitement of the phenomenal experience of watching the daring feat of the divers plummeting into the deep narrow gorges from incredible heights. It was as if a heavy cloud hung over the remainder of our trip. My positivity was forced, and Jim had retreated into a place of suspicion and quiet, impenetrable solitude.

Thankfully, there were no more dramatic occurrences. We stayed on the ship each remaining day of the cruise, never venturing too far from our cabin so Jim could take seclusion and rest when needed. The highlight of our day revolved around the delicious cuisine we partook of in the various restaurants on the ship, but even though the food was wonderful, we dined in a strained state of silence most of the time. Jim seemed unable to shake off the irrational paranoia he felt, and I could not penetrate the wall that had gone up between us. My prayer each night was that we could make it through the following day safely and without upset.

The day of disembarking the ship was finally here. I knew we were going to have to use a wheelchair to accomplish this big feat. I had finished our packing the evening before and put out our big suitcases in the hallway for the porters to gather very early the next day. I knew Jim would never agree to the wheelchair, so I picked up the phone in our room and asked for one to be delivered to our room before the time we were scheduled to depart. I knew for his protection I had to make the decision myself, even if it meant he would be unhappy and resistant.

He objected immediately after I hung up the phone just as I knew he would. I kindly told him how the next couple of hours were going to involve us standing and walking continuously off the ship and through the airport, including going through customs. We were on a limited schedule and had to make sure we got on our flight in time. The chair was the only way we would be able to make it.

I silently prayed he wouldn't get angry and insist on walking as he had done in Acapulco. There were just too many connections and processes we had to go through. The responsibility of dealing with the tickets and customs and luggage and transportation to the airport was all mine. I was all too keenly aware of this fact. Yes, our lives were shifting and changing rapidly, and I had to keep constantly pushing back the fear. Today, I had to not just take it one day at a time, but one hour and even one minute. And I had to ask for help when I needed it, not only from God but from anyone else I could find.

When the wheelchair arrived at our cabin, Jim regarded it with scorn. "I'm not getting in that chair. I can walk just fine!"

My worst fears were coming true. "I know you can walk, but we may have to wait for a long time in lines, and there may not be places you can find to sit and rest. With the wheelchair we can put our carry-on bags in your lap so I can retrieve our big suitcases at the dock and get them to the van to go to the airport. People will help us if you're in the chair, and we're going to need help!"

About three hours later, we arrived at Gate B35 ready to board our flight for the lengthy trip home. My nerves were frazzled, and I could see that my husband was completely exhausted. I wondered if he realized we would never have made it without the wheelchair. Or was he still dwelling in the unhappy, resentful frame of mind with which he had begun this interminably long day? He had finally sat down in the chair when our color was called to depart the ship.

The chair did make a difference, as the attendant had called us to the front of the line when he saw us waiting. We still had an extended wait outside the ship in the hot California sun as our line snaked across a covered walkway and on the outside edge of the large building on the dock, where we showed our cruise ID for the final time. After going through the massive luggage area and finally spotting the suitcases with the brightly-colored yarn tags we had attached, I asked the first person I saw with a name tag where we could acquire the assistance to get our luggage from there to our airport transport service. We had to give up the chair at the van, but our luggage was loaded, and we managed to get our small bags on and find a seat.

At the airport, I was shocked to observe a sea of people standing outside the building, just waiting to go inside. We both had to stand in an unshaded, slow-moving line. It was midday, and the sun was directly overhead, baking our heads for about a half-hour. Pulling our big bags along with the smaller ones stacked on top, it was awkward and tiring.

Finally, we were inside the building, and again I searched the area for a person with a name tag. At this point, we had to go through customs, then head to the luggage and check-in area. There was no objection to sitting in the chair this time, and the attendant pushed him all the way across the airport and into the elevator to the upper area to our boarding gate. Although I had allowed for what I thought was more than sufficient time to make our flight, we had barely made it. The first group of travelers were already beginning to check in, and the attendant pushed us right up to the front of the line. At the entrance to the plane, an airline attendant found us seats near the front, and at long last, we could take a deep breath and relax.

We still had one change of planes before arriving back to Kansas City, where our son would be waiting to pick us up. Thankfully the biggest part of the long ordeal was behind us. Within a few minutes of boarding, Jim was sound asleep, but the adrenalin was still coursing through my mind. Once again, I felt the burden of all the responsibility being squarely placed on my shoulders. I had been the one keeping track of all the papers; the customs forms, the boarding passes, the passports, credit cards, and cash for the tips.

Again, I realized that during this trip, a big change had transpired. It was very difficult to keep from letting my personal emotions take over. I was mad; I was exhausted; and I was resentful. But as I leaned back in my seat and closed my eyes, a realization hit me squarely in the face. I couldn't be angry with my husband or resentful of his thoughts or actions. It wasn't his fault. It wasn't HIM making those irrational accusations or demands. It was my new, biggest, number one enemy called CANCER, and we were only beginning the hard part of the battle.

It would probably be the biggest challenge I might ever have to deal with. So, I better get ready and I better be strong and tough. Because, although I knew our adversary was going to ultimately win the battle for Jim's earthly mind and body, he would not win the victory over his soul. And I would, with God's help, still be standing strong and faithful in the end.

Chapter 25
The Second Haven

Late April, 2011

THE NEXT FEW DAYS AFTER we arrived back in Emporia, Kansas were somewhat foggy. We both slept extra hours to catch up from the fatigue we felt from the cruise. I was thankful we had made it safely back without having to receive any medical help on the entire trip. I knew we were divinely protected and realized Jim could have easily had a bad fall from the dizziness he had experienced. I thought about what might have happened had an accident occurred in a foreign country.

As I reflected on the new phase we were entering, I was strongly directed to make a change in our living arrangements. I felt impressed it was time to leave our son's home and find a place of our own where Jim could experience peace and privacy. Although I had no idea how difficult the next few months could be, I believed we needed to be close to our extended family for support, and in an environment close to medical care if needed.

After discussing this prospect with my sister one day, she generously offered to let us stay with her and her husband until we found a house. The prospect was appealing, as Jim and my brother-in-law had always gotten along well, and right now I needed the emotional support they could give me during this transitional phase we were experiencing. With the Lord's timing and guidance, I was sure He had a plan to provide for our needs, just as He had been faithful to provide for us so far.

Leaving our son's home with only a few personal items, and a variety of clothes which would fit into two large suitcases, I felt the peace that comes when you are obedient to follow the Lord's leading hand. Our son had provided exactly what we had needed the past five months, and I will always be grateful for the way he had opened wide his arms to us. We would only be moving a couple of hours away from him, so we could still see him and our grandchildren at regular intervals.

Shortly after settling in at my sister's house, one of my first priorities was to find a local doctor for Jim. Someone who would be familiar with his medical history and could assist us with what lay before us. This town also had a good hospital. In talking with my sis and brother-in-law, I also decided I needed to check into hospice care. There was a local office downtown, and I made an appointment to explore what it was all about.

The lady in the office was genuinely compassionate and explained how their services operated. In order to receive their services, I had to get a signed referral from two doctors to recommend hospice care and to state it was needed. When we arrived at the internal medicine doctor's office, I presented him with Jim's prognosis records and described what treatment he had received in Oklahoma.

He wanted a complete blood panel analysis, and as we visited with him, I asked if he could help us get into hospice care. After examining Jim and asking him a variety of questions, he requested we return in a few days to go over his blood test results. Then he would decide if he felt we needed hospice. I would call his doctor in Oklahoma to be his other reference.

We had gone back to the treatment center for the three-month and then six-month follow-up MRIs. At the three-month check-up, our treatment physician had told us the tumor was about the same as when Jim had left the center, but he expected it to begin to grow again rapidly and there would not be any further treatments he could do. Sure enough, the six-month MRI had shown some regrowth. We were sad yet realistic about the news. We had known he could not receive more radiation.

At the second appointment, the local doctor showed us how several of the results of the workup were either too low or too high. I was anxious to take the results home with me and compare them to the ones from his last testing. But without hesitation, he stated he would refer us to hospice.

It was concerning that he so readily agreed, and even more so when I called the lady at hospice to tell her he would refer us. She flatly stated that this doctor had very rarely referred anyone to them. It was another confirmation to me that Jim's condition was rapidly changing, and this was the right course for us to take.

After filling out the paperwork and giving her a complete medication list of prescriptions that he was taking, she gave me an informational pamphlet on what the hospice program was all about and answered all of my many questions. The paperwork would be processed, and she expected us to be approved within a couple of weeks. Once again, I felt assured we were on the right path. I was determined to grant my husband's wishes about avoiding hospitals and other medical facilities in his last stages of life, caring for him at home as long as humanly possible. Now that I had the hospice people to help me, I felt I could possibly make that goal a reality.

I had a big decision to make about housing. I didn't want to impose upon my sister for very long, but I didn't know if this town would be my permanent place to live after I lost my husband. Therefore, purchasing a home there might be a mistake. I felt like we needed a simple, small residence for the time being, but this town had very few rental houses available. My prayer was a request for clear direction as to which path to take. In the meantime, we started looking at the houses for sale in town.

As we scanned the local newspaper, there was one place that caught Jim's eye. It was located a few miles from town and had some acreage for lease along with the house. Of course, we had lived in the country most all our married years, and I understood how it would be more appealing for him to choose a rural setting.

Reluctantly, I agreed to go drive out for a look at the place. The home looked beautiful, a one-story brick ranch style, but the price was not in our budget. When I told him it was too expensive, he explained how we might be able to afford it if he was able to farm the acreage and get money from the crops. Another moment of hard reality. There was, of course, no way he would ever be able to farm again, but his mind had not accepted that fact. There were many more times ahead when I realized in so many ways Jim had not accepted the truth about his condition.

I learned hope comes in many forms, and squelching that hope was not always the wise choice to make. I had to be extra sensitive to words that I used during those delicate circumstances when my husband would talk about the future. I prayed for extra insight and wisdom during those difficult moments.

I also recalled how our doctor in OKC had warned us about this stage of regrowth of the tumor. He had recounted to us how one patient had spent an exorbitant amount of money on an unreasonable purchase without consulting his wife. Another patient had gone to his bank, withdrawn the majority of his savings, and given it away to a distant relative.

I remembered the day at my son's house when Jim was determined to go out and purchase a brand-new red SUV, although ours was just fine and finally paid off. The car salesman had continued to call us every few days, even after we moved away from the town, encouraging us to make the deal. I finally had to bluntly tell him we were not shopping for a new car. Period.

My sister and brother-in-law were wonderful during this transition time. I had exactly the support and encouragement I so desperately needed. Charlie would take Jim out for drives in the country to look at the crops around the area or by the John Deere dealership to check out all the farm equipment they had on the lot. I had my sis to confide in, and both to sound ideas off of.

During those weeks, Jim began to experience more incidents of both physical and mental changes. He began to experience times of loss of balance and weakness in his legs. He would get up from a chair, walk down the hallway toward the bathroom, and suddenly start to lose his balance. When this happened, one of us would run to where he was with a portable stool we kept handy to put under his legs so that he could sit down for a few minutes until the dizziness subsided.

One time, as he was turning into the bathroom from the hall, I saw him begin to sway and knew he was going to fall. I ran to help him, at the same time calling for Charlie to bring the stool. As he started falling toward me, I tried to catch him to hold him upright, but this time he continued to fall over, and before I knew it, I was on the floor underneath him. My left thumb was jammed down at an awkward angle from the other fingers, and it throbbed with pain. But thankfully, neither of us was badly hurt. At six-foot-two and weighing over two hundred pounds, my husband was not easy to hold up.

After this incident of realizing the danger of him falling, I knew we needed to find a walker for him to use to keep him safe, as these times of imbalance were starting to occur on a regular basis. There were days when everything seemed normal, and we would laugh and talk about our many years of family experiences together. Jim and Charlie would sit and watch western shows and movies on TV, and Lin and I would talk and cook and do other household tasks together. What a relief it was to be able to have their support and love in the good days and the more difficult ones when we had to deal with some of the increasing symptoms of Jim's condition.

Besides my sis, my mom and Jim's dad and handicapped sister also lived in this same town. Jim's dad was aging, and it was becoming more difficult for him to care for his daughter, who had become brain-damaged several years before in a tragic hospital incident. He had cared for her by himself after Jim's mom passed away suddenly, and recently they had made the decision to move to Wichita, Kansas, to reside in an assisted living facility.

One day we were over at his house visiting them, and Jim's dad asked us what we were planning to do about our housing situation. I told him we were looking around to see what was available to buy or rent in town, and Jim asked him what he was planning to do with his house once they moved. He said he would probably be listing it with an agent, and Jim asked him if he would consider selling his house to us.

Suddenly, Jim's dad looked at us and emphatically said, "Well, no, I wouldn't sell the house to you, but by God, I will give it to you!"

Had I just heard what I thought I'd heard? Was he saying he wanted to GIVE us his house? I felt my face become flushed, and I looked at Jim in wonder.

"Dad, you can't give us your house. We could pay you for it, but it would be a great help to us, since we need a place of our own to live in. We can't impose on Barb's sister much longer, and we haven't been able to find a place so far."

"This would save me all the hassle of trying to sell it or rent it out and dealing with it from Wichita by phone. This would solve your problem and mine, too. This would be a great relief to me, and I want to help you, too. You and Barb have helped us out so many times over the years, like when your mom had her kidney operation, and Barb came and stayed with us a month.

"Also, she was here to help when your mom passed away. I want to do this for you, and since it is paid for, all we need to do is call my lawyer and get it transferred over to your name. In fact, I'll set up an appointment right now so we can get it taken care of before we leave to go to Wichita."

"Are you sure about this?" I asked him. "Do you need some more time to think about it? I can't believe you are offering to give us a house!"

"I'm sure," he said with certainty. "We have never helped you out before, and now I have the chance to do it, and I want to!"

Another miracle in the string of miracles we had experienced since this journey had begun. I wanted to leap for joy and start praising God for His outpouring of blessings He continued to give us amidst the great pain and uncertainty we were living in.

The very next day we owned a house, and within a few weeks, we moved in. Because we needed to do some cosmetic repairs and add a walk-in shower for Jim to be able to use, I had several people to schedule in to perform the needed repairs. It was amazing how quickly and easily it came together.

This confirmed again we were in God's will. Charlie got busy building a wheelchair ramp from our front door to the sidewalk, and my precious friend Donna offered to paint the entire inside of the house (which she did all by herself, refusing to accept any payment for her labor). Because Jim's sister required handicap bars, we did not have to install any.

By moving day, we had a new walk-in shower, new carpet in the bedrooms, fresh paint on the walls, new flooring in the kitchen-dining room area, and several other improvements. My son from Texas came up and mounted a large-screen TV on the wall of the room where Jim could comfortably watch his favorite westerns from the bed he would eventually spend most of his time in.

In preparation of our move into a much smaller house than we had lived in when we were in New Mexico, we purchased a big storage shed to hold the remainder of our belongings. We needed a very uncrowded, clutter-free, simple home for now; one which would allow free movement throughout.

Jim began to be obsessed with getting his farm pickup moved down from our son's house. He often asked when we were going to make the trip back up to his house to get it. When the subject would come up, I usually tried to change the subject or tactfully put off his requests. It was no longer possible to even consider him being able to drive it, and I felt good knowing it was safely stored two hours away. I had hoped that 'out of sight' would eventually produce 'out of mind.' I totally understood his desire.

That truck represented much more than a means of transportation to him. It embodied the identity of who he was, who he had been for most of his life. It represented all the years when he had been the hard-working, capable, respected, superman farmer with endless energy and extensive capabilities to solve every problem that arose. This was another example of allowing my husband to keep his hope alive.

I realized more and more the delicate balance of hope and despair. Hope encouraged the will to live, despair produced depression and loss of will. And safety frequently battled with hope. I often found myself in the middle between the two, having to make hard decisions.

Finally, Charlie accompanied me to rent a wheelchair; safety had to take precedence over pride. Jim had narrowly escaped serious injury several times with his balance episodes. The many bruises on his arms and legs were proof. The acceptance of the chair naturally produced a certain loss of dignity, but also obtained the desired level of safety.

One of the hardest days of conflict over the pickup arrived a few days before we moved into the house. Charlie had planned on taking Jim on a much-needed outing away from the confines of the house. The plan was to travel the fifty miles to the business which was building our new storage shed and inspect it for delivery in the next few days. As soon as they were headed out of town, Jim told Charlie they needed to go on to Emporia and he would drive his pickup back.

Charlie very nicely told Jim they couldn't do it this day as they were headed to look at the storage shed. Jim would not change the subject, but insisted Charlie take him on up to get the truck. The situation continued to elevate until Jim finally demanded that Charlie stop the vehicle as he wanted OUT. Not knowing what else to do, Charlie turned his pickup around and headed back home with Jim sulking all the way.

To make matters worse, when they arrived back at the house, Charlie hurriedly got out and came in to let me know what was going on. As I approached the truck to talk to Jim, I found he had locked the doors with the keys still inside. No persuasion would get him to unlock the doors, so I called my oldest son and asked him if he would call Jim's cell phone and try to talk to him. I helplessly stood outside as I heard Jim's phone ring. Although I wasn't sure what was said, after several minutes, Jim got off the phone and continued to sit there, staring straight ahead.

At last, I heard the clicking of the door locks. He slowly got out of the truck and somehow made it inside on his own, going straight to the bedroom we were sleeping in. I stayed outside and took some long, deep breaths. Once again, I reminded myself it was the cancer messing with my husband's logic.

A few days before our move, we were shopping in Walmart for some food and personal care items. Jim had decided to come along, and I had persuaded him to sit in one of their wheelchairs during the long jaunt through the store. Pushing him from one section of the store to the next to find various items, Jim said he wanted to go back to the sporting goods area of the store. Not thinking anything about it, I asked him which aisle he wanted to look at.

"I want to go over by the checkout area and look for a twenty-two."

"A gun?" I asked him quizzically.

"Yes, I want to find a gun to give to Charlie. I want to give him something for helping us out the past few weeks, and to thank him for building the ramp over at the house."

As soon as the words came out, my antennae of suspicion went up. Lately, Jim had been getting very discouraged about his condition. He had asked me several times what we were going to do next to help him get over his cancer. He kept telling me to find another doctor or treatment center that would get him better. At times, he would even get angry, and accuse me that I didn't care. Those were hurtful and delicate situations, when I would try to assure him we had gotten the best treatment available.

I would always remind him the trials and other alternative treatments would most likely take us far away from family into hospital environments. This was directly opposite of what he had expressed he wanted to do. Those conversations would seem to satisfy him for a few days, then the anxiousness would resurface again. I knew during these depressive days when he felt his strength and control lessoning, irrational thoughts were likely to surface.

My sis was a couple of aisles away, and I left Jim to rapidly fill her in on what was going on. She grasped the situation quickly, and immediately went up to Jim.

"Barb says you want to get Charlie something. I know exactly what that could be. He's been talking about wanting one of those Coleman camping lanterns with the bright LED lighting. I think they have them over here a few aisles away."

I got behind the wheelchair and started pushing him toward the camping supplies.

"Yes, here's just what he's been wanting." She picked up the lantern from the shelf.

"This is perfect!" I eagerly took the lantern and placed it into our basket.

"Well, if that's really what you think he would want," Jim reluctantly stated. "But we were talking the other day about how he had always wanted a 22 rifle and never got one growing up."

Maybe it was true. Maybe he really wanted to get the gun for Charlie. But my gut instinct said otherwise. I guess I will never know for sure, but it was another instance where I had to gravitate toward the matter of safety.

Chapter 26
The Mysterious Walk

May, 2011

AT LAST, WE WERE SETTLED in our own private space in our own home. We had moved into another stage of our journey. Jim had finally surrendered to the wheelchair when out of bed, but still had enough mobility to get from the bed to the chair and into the bathroom with assistance of the walker. The wonderful hospice team arrived to make our transitions go as easily as possible, ready to provide safety aides and much-needed advice. It was so reassuring knowing they were only a call away. The nurse visited our house once a week and would come more often as needed. Included in their service, a chaplain came to visit us, offering prayer and a listening ear.

Friends we had met brought meals and offered help in any way we needed. One sweet lady brought over crushed fine ice at least once or twice a week. Such a small gift, but what a caring service, as Jim enjoyed it with a cold drink in those hot summer days. A couple of people came over and finished painting the trim in the room with the new shower. Old friends from Jim's high school days stopped by for short visits, and many family members came, providing support and love.

With the help of hospice, I had decided we would ease up on the strict regimen of diet and supplements we had diligently followed for months. Although I still kept stringent records of blood sugar levels, I wanted to allow Jim to enjoy whatever food and drink he desired at this time. When we discussed this, the first thing he requested was buttered popcorn from the movie theater, and real cherry coke. Different family members would make a special trip to the theater just to buy him his popcorn. It brought a smile to his face every time!

As the days went by, the one big source of unhappiness still stemmed from the feeling Jim had that I was not doing enough to find a cure for his cancer. From the time of diagnosis, Jim clung desperately to life, often expressing how he wanted to be around to see his grandchildren grow up. After bringing it up again one day, I finally decided to call our doctor from the cancer treatment center we had gone to and discuss the matter with him.

"He just can't accept there is nothing further we can do," I told him. "The only thing I could think of was to ask you if maybe you could talk to him. Perhaps he would believe it if the words came from you. I know he respects you."

"There really isn't any more treatment that would help Jim at this point. The last MRI back in January showed the tumor was twenty percent larger than right after the treatments. We cannot give him any more radiation. If you would like, I will tell him this." It was a very sad moment, and I could tell the doctor didn't want to tell Jim this any more than I did.

I took the phone and told Jim his doctor from Oklahoma was on the phone and wanted to visit with him.

I only heard Jim's end of the conversation, but I could tell the doctor was explaining the situation to him. I fought back tears as Jim sat there with the phone up to his ear, listening intently.

"And there's nothing else out there, maybe in another state?" I heard him ask.

Whatever the doctor said did not make Jim happy. When he finally laid down the phone, he sat there with his eyes closed for a long time.

After giving him some time, I went over and hugged him long and hard. There was really nothing else to say but I was there for him, would do anything I could for him, and I loved him. Not long after this, for the first time since he was diagnosed, he said the words out loud.

"I'm not going to make it, am I?"

I thought my heart would break in two.

During these difficult days, another miracle came by phone one day. Since leaving the treatment center, I had received no billing statement concerning the amount we would still owe after the insurance company paid their part. It remained a big question mark I wasn't sure I wanted to know the answer to. Amidst all the challenges that were constantly occurring in our lives, I had filed the matter into the back recesses of my mind.

One day, it hit me that months had passed by, and in order to plan for our financial future, I needed to find out the dollar amount we would have to still be liable for. I had left a message on Peggy's phone, not knowing the direct number to the business office. The next afternoon, she returned my call with amazing news. After discussing the matter with her superiors, it had been decided the facility would write off the balance of our account, and we owed nothing at all.

I really could not believe my ears! When would these provisions of magnanimous proportions end? I know I must have asked her several times before I was convinced it was true. With God, there evidently were no limits to His goodness toward us. I got off the phone, rejoicing for the remainder of the day, and catching myself shaking my head in wonder several times.

Later in August of that year, I unexpectedly received a check through the mail from the insurance company in New Mexico for $100. No explanation, no memo at the bottom. I wasn't even going to try to figure it out. For some reason, it struck me as humorous. I just had to share this with my friend Peggy, who also found it hilarious. The irony of it all . . . .

One of my husband's best friends called to check on Jim. During the conversation, he asked me for a big favor.

"Barb, can you assure me that during these rough days you won't walk out on Jim and leave him?"

I was shocked he could even ask such a question.

"Of course. Why would you ask me this?" I replied quickly.

"Because I know that some people just can't handle such hard circumstances. They feel that they can't deal with the situation, and they walk away. I've known people to do that, and I want to know that you won't do this to my friend."

I had never even entertained such a thought. Now that he brought it up, I had known one situation in my husband's family where that very thing had happened. When Jim's sister suffered the damage to her brain and became handicapped, her husband of only a couple of years left her because he couldn't handle it. It was devastating for her on top of everything else she was going through. I guess people do those sorts of drastic acts when they feel helpless and overwhelmed.

"I thought you knew me better than that. I can promise you I will be with Jim to the end. Yes, it's harder than I ever imagined it would be, but I'm here to see it through."

"I'm so relieved to hear you say this. I just had to ask, because I care so much for Jim."

In a way, it made me angry, but ultimately, I was thankful my husband had such a caring friend who would look out for him enough to ask.

People could be great, and some people could be so insensitive! One day a pastor came over for a visit. After a few moments of small talk, he sat in the living-room chair, and leaned forward intently.

"Jim, what is the most important thing you've ever done in your life?" he asked directly.

I had awakened Jim from a nap when the man had unexpectedly arrived at our front door. At this point, he was sleeping several hours in the afternoons, and it took a while for him to clear his groggy mind.

After several awkward moments of hesitation, Jim briefly raised his head up and replied, "Well, I guess it would be the day I married her." He glanced quickly in my direction.

"Oh, okay, well what else? Would there be any other decision that you made that was important?" Jim could tell the man had not been satisfied with his first answer.

"Well, it was when I had my three boys." He looked to see if that was the answer the man wanted. It obviously was not.

The man sternly looked at Jim, and loudly started quoting a Scripture verse at him.

I quickly responded, "Jim is a Christian and has served the Lord for many years. He has been a deacon, a Sunday school teacher, an AWANA leader and has led many people to the Lord!"

What was I doing? I had felt like I had to convince this man that Jim was a believer by listing his credentials. I could sense Jim's insecurity and confusion. If this man, as a pastor, knew he was living in an advanced stage of brain cancer, surely, he would realize this was not the time to use this intimidating, condemning type of approach. Obviously, he lacked true compassion and was on some sort of mission. It brought out my defensiveness for my husband, knowing Jim's mind was not working correctly, and at this time what he needed was gentle love and compassion. I abruptly thanked the man for coming by, told him Jim needed his rest, and ended the visit as quickly as I could.

"Did I do okay? Did I answer the questions right?" Jim nervously asked as soon as the door closed. I could tell he was disturbed and confused.

"Yes, honey, you did just fine. You gave good answers." I was livid, realizing the visit had caused such distress. I learned another lesson that day. True love and compassion for people always triumphs over legalistic, judgmental religious passion. People, even those with a damaged brain, pick up on the difference. The man never returned to check on Jim's condition again, and I was very relieved for that favor.

Even as I experienced the advancing effects of this cruel invasion on Jim's body, there were still moments of clarity of thought, and I was thankful for each of these precious memories.

One day, out of the blue, Jim brought up the subject of the strange experience on the cruise. "I just want you to know that I'm sorry about how I acted that night. I don't know what I was thinking, but now I realize that I was totally wrong. I wasn't thinking right. It seemed so real at the time, but now I know it wasn't."

This was such an unexpected blessing in the midst of the norm which now mainly consisted of irrationality, short-term memory loss, and long periods of silence. I clung to these moments like a drowning person clings to a life preserver.

Gradually, the part of the brain that told the legs how to move was completely captured by the cancer. Walking became impossible and transferring Jim from the bed to his portable potty or into the wheelchair and into his shower chair became more and more difficult. He always thought he could do those things for himself, but it wasn't true. The hospice nurses showed me ways to maneuver my body and his to achieve these increasingly difficult necessary movements. Thankfully, I was physically strong from the many years of working hard and doing consistent exercise in the high altitudes of New Mexico. His large frame presented a big challenge, but I was still determined to handle his care at home where he wanted to be.

One night toward the end of June, a few weeks after he had completely lost the function of his legs, a strange event took place. The day had been long and difficult, and I quickly fell into a deep, exhausted sleep beside my husband. I was on the side of the bed against the wall, while he lay next to the open side of the room, close to the portable potty chair, with the door to the bedroom a few feet away.

As impulsive thinking had become more common, I always closed the door to the hallway in case Jim might wake up during the night and try to get up by himself. I had also placed pillows directly by his side of the bed in case he might accidentally roll out.

After several hours of deep sleep, I slowly woke up and prepared myself for another long day of caretaking. I rolled over toward my husband's side, wondering if he was awake yet. To my great surprise, his side of the bed was empty. Jumping up, I ran around the bed, expecting to find him on the floor, but to my growing amazement, there was no trace of him.

As I whirled around to face the door, I saw it standing wide open, and frantically ran down the hall quickly looking through each doorway. Straight down the hallway at the back of the house through the den, a small door opened into the attached garage. Right outside the door, two concrete steps led down into the floor of the garage. That door was also wide open. My mind raced to think what could have happened. But my husband was not there either.

Backing up, I went through the other door from the den which led into the small bathroom, through the laundry room, and into the kitchen in the front of the house. After finding no trace of him, I went rapidly from the kitchen into the long living room, and there, soundly sleeping with his head on the crossbar of the maple end table, was my husband. He was lying on his stomach with his head turned to one side against the hard-wooden bar.

"Jim, wake up! What in the world are you doing here?" My heart was still racing. Slowly, as he groaned and tried to turn over to look at me, I inspected his body for signs of injury. Should I call an ambulance? He must have fallen to the carpeted floor. To my amazement, I could find no bruises or obvious signs of bodily damage.

"Are you hurting anywhere? Can you sit up?"

"I'm okay. But I do need some help to get up," he calmly said.

It was one thing to help someone move from one object to another, but it was another thing to bring a large man from the floor all the way up to a wheelchair. It was important I stay fit and uninjured to continue in my role as a caretaker. I needed help, and now was the time to ask for it. I called the hospice number and quickly described the situation. Within a few minutes, a male nurse arrived, and we got Jim into the wheelchair and back to the bedroom safely. He seemed exhausted and slept for several hours afterward.

As I discussed the event with the hospice nurse, he was astounded. He said he had never heard of anyone who had lost control of his legs be able to ever regain that ability. When Jim's regular hospice worker came a couple of days later, I related the episode to her. She too, was completely astounded and was anxious to talk to the doctor and hear what he would say. I told her it wasn't just a few steps, but because of the evidence of the open doors throughout the house, he had walked the complete length of the house and circled back around to the living room. Thank God he had not tried to step out into the garage, or he could have been severely injured. What was he trying to do, or what had he been searching for?

I hoped I would get some answers from Jim when he woke up. But to my dismay, he didn't seem to remember what had happened or didn't want to talk about it. After talking the situation over with the hospice doctor, the nurse confirmed what she had stated. Once gone, the use of the legs could not have returned from a physiological aspect.

Questions continued to flash in my mind. *How could he have possibly gotten out of bed, through the pillows on the floor, and out the door of our bedroom without making a noise which would have immediately awakened me?*

For the past few weeks, he had not even been able to get up out of bed by himself. And the journey throughout the rest of the house? It was a big mystery that didn't seem to have an explanation. It was the one and only time the use of his legs returned.

Chapter 27
The Healing

Late June, 2011

A FEW DAYS LATER, Jim's very best friend from western Kansas came to visit him. Jim was so happy to see him and loved hearing all about the latest news from his farm. During the years we were neighbors, the two of them had developed a deep friendship. They were not just neighbors who loved to talk about farming together. They were bound by their common faith and values.

Toward the end of his visit, his friend asked Jim some pointed questions about how he had been doing. To my great surprise, Jim looked directly at him and said, "I know this sounds strange, but I've been healed."

Since the discussion on the phone with his doctor, Jim had quit asking me to pursue other avenues of treatment. He seemed to accept his condition instead of constantly struggling against it. His increased loss of function in many areas had gradually increased, but it didn't bring on the deep depression like it had before.

The progression of the tumor was obvious to anyone who came around. At times, Jim seemed to live in the past, asking me when our youngest son would be home from school, and when his next baseball or basketball game was scheduled so we could go watch him play. This made him anxious at times, and the only thing that seemed to help was a phone call from Josh himself, explaining to his dad he was doing well and working in a job in a different state. Jim was sleeping more and more during the daytime and would be silent for long lengths of time.

"That's wonderful, Jim!" his friend replied.

"I can't explain it, but I know that I am healed," he reiterated.

This was new to me. He hadn't said anything about such a thing before, but I could see the certainty in his eyes. I was so thankful Jim's friend had replied in affirmation. Somehow, there had been a transformation from depression and dread of his impending death to the peace and certainty of healing. What caused this change? Had it happened the night of his 'walk'? Had the Lord shown him a glimpse of his future where he would once again be healthy and whole? I guess I won't have those answers here, but someday in heaven I can't wait to find out.

The long, steaming hot days of summer continued to tick off. July arrived, and I had learned well the lesson of taking one day at a time. Extra measure of strength and patience and faith were doled out to me daily. My son from Texas came up for three weeks to help me care for his dad. Being six-foot-four inches tall and strongly built, he was a tremendous boost both physically and emotionally.

I could discuss the incidents of the day with him, and Jim loved having him there. Jim had lost control over some more of his bodily functions, and new and unpleasant tasks were added to our list of caretaking duties, but Chad took them in stride. He was a Sports

Medicine Trainer and had much knowledge and compassion in health matters. And besides, this was his dad. He would have done anything for him, and I was grateful beyond words for his help.

The hospice care team had brought in a hospital bed, which made it easier to get Jim in and out of bed. We put it up in the back-den area of the house where it was quiet and restful. There he could watch TV and take long naps without being disturbed by other noises in the front part of the house.

One hot afternoon, one of Jim's best buddies from high school came over to visit. He brought along a gift from other fellow members of the football team Jim had played on. The football was signed by almost all the team, and as Wayne presented it to Jim, he choked up with tears. For a few minutes the two friends reminisced together about the carefree, wonderful days of youth when their biggest care was beating their rival team, and deciding how they would celebrate together afterwards.

This small class, which consisted of many more boys than girls, had bonded together with strong friendships which had lasted throughout the many years since graduation. Their relationships were rare and special, and when they got together, their high school stories always resulted in hours of boisterous laughter! This visit was priceless for Jim, and for the first time in many months, I heard him laugh out loud. Cancer was beaten that day, and inwardly I rejoiced over the brief victory.

As I saw the advancement of the disease increasing, I made several phone calls and arranged for most of the family to come together for a special visit. As in most families, ours had a few broken relationships, and those differences increasingly bothered Jim. He repeatedly told me during the few moments of alertness how much he wanted to see forgiveness and reconciliation between these family members.

On that special weekend, he spoke to each person separately and privately, asking them to grant his final wishes. It was very emotional for several people that day, with many tears shed and promises made. I am happy to say most of those promises were followed through on, and there have been some broken relationships repaired. Score another victory over cancer!

As time moved forward, Jim seemed to withdraw into himself a little more each day. His appetite decreased. He couldn't even be tempted with movie butter-flavored popcorn beyond a few bites. He still loved sipping his cherry coke, but mostly his meals were picked at rather than eaten. Periods of sleep became longer and more frequent, and he barely spoke when he was awake. I found myself sleeping more frequently on the couch across the room from his hospital bed instead of in the bedroom down the hall.

Often, I would sit and read Scripture aloud to him and pray out loud for all our loved ones far and near. He seemed to be at complete peace during those special moments, and although he wouldn't voice his approval, sometimes he would open his eyes and reach for my hand.

Sometimes, as I lay on the couch listening to him breathe, tears would continually and silently roll down my cheeks. I didn't want him to know that I was crying. He had always disliked crying. Perhaps he just didn't know how to handle a crying woman, but throughout our long years of marriage, he had always become agitated at my tears. Right or wrong, it was just the way it was, and I knew it probably stemmed from the concept taught early that strong people don't cry.

Although Jim had mellowed out much over the years, and I had even seen tears spring to his eyes when he was touched deeply by something, I instinctively knew that what he needed now was strength and positive confidence from me. There would be time for crying later.

The hospice nurses came as I needed them to, and on their visits I would take advantage of their vast past experiences by asking them endless questions, which they patiently answered. What would happen at the end? How would I know that it was getting near? The male nurse patiently explained how I would be able to recognize various stages toward the end, especially concerning the types of breathing that would come.

After testing his oxygen level one day, he suggested that setting up oxygen by the hospital bed might make Jim more comfortable. He also reminded me that at the first sign of discomfort or pain, they could provide pain meds immediately. Their goal was to help the family deal with death in the best possible way with loving acts of kindness and compassion. I can testify to the successful achievement of that goal through my personal experience. Their support and expertise were invaluable to me, and I couldn't have achieved Jim's wishes without them.

My son's family from Texas was visiting, and once again I was deeply grateful for their love and support. All my sons had visited when they could, and each time they came I was greatly encouraged. Jim loved their visits. Now that there were few waking hours with Jim, I had more time to realistically think about the necessary preparations to be made.

One morning I drove the few miles to the funeral home I had decided to use for Jim's funeral care. Although it was difficult to make these necessary arrangements, I felt it would be better to do it now than during the extremely emotional hours after death occurred. In preparing all the details ahead of time, I would know exactly what to do when the hour came.

I had a phone number and a name of a person to call who would immediately come to assist me. I was spared the practical decisions of colors and quality and pricing when shock would take over my mind in the hours immediately following the death of my loved one. In these long days of feeling helpless to stop the advancement of the disease, there was something practical I could do, and it was such a relief to me.

I called our long-time friend and pastor from western Kansas to see if he would be willing to perform the funeral. No one else could give a eulogy about Jim the way Larry could. He had worshipped, talked, played, and gone through many life events with our family. Our sons had grown up and gone through college together as best friends. We had spent countless hours together at their home and at the church. He immediately agreed to preach Jim's funeral.

Not only was he our friend, but I knew him to be especially gifted when it came to funerals. He had a special way of honoring the memory of the deceased with beautiful personal accounts of their life. I also knew he would emphasize the importance of knowing and having a personal relationship with the Lord. Accomplishing these important arrangements brought peace and relief to my mind.

Thankfully, Jim was not experiencing much pain at all. The oxygen allowed him to comfortably sleep without the aid of the sleep apnea mask he had worn for the past couple of years. I could now barely get him to swallow a few bites of soft food or sip a little water from a straw during the brief moments he was awake.

The hospice nurses encouraged me to give him only what he would take and not force him to eat or drink. He was off most of his diabetic meds as he could no longer swallow the pills. I would still administer his insulin shot daily to his stomach area. This seemed to be the only time he reacted with a grimace or a moan.

It became hard to tell when he was awake, as he rarely spoke or made a sound at all. Occasionally I would see him move his hand or briefly blink his eyes, and I would offer him a sip of water and talk to him for a little while. Most of the time there was no response.

On the twenty-ninth of July, he began to exhibit short bursts of breaths followed by long even ones. I recognized this as one of the patterns of breathing I would see as the end drew near. The hospice nurse came at my call and told me this was perfectly normal during this time. She said he could stay in this pattern for a few days or less. After checking all his vitals and making sure he was comfortable and stable, she squeezed my hand and told me to call her as often as I wanted. She would be there within a few minutes time.

Although my brain told me the time was near, I suddenly could not accept what all the signs were telling me. I had somehow arrived at my own conclusion that Jim would stay with us until November or December. *Wasn't that the end of the two years since the Lord had spoken to him?*

I had to remind myself he had been told two years or less, and the appointed time was apparently very near. Several people had told me that even when you know death is coming, you are still not ready for it when it arrives. I affirmed this truth now.

My son and family were in the house with me, and I explained the breathing patterns to them, stating it could be a few days or sooner. As we continued to care for Jim's personal cleanliness and basic needs, we all seemed to be holding our own collective breaths. I slept fitfully that night on the couch beside Jim, waking every few minutes to listen for his breathing.

I prayed and asked God to give me and my family the strength to endure and remain calm in our time of waiting. I asked Him to draw near to Jim and put His loving arms around him as he prepared to leave this earthly life. Time passed slowly as I heard the clock slowly ticking by the seconds in the quiet night hours. I heard the air conditioner click off and on in its cycle, working to control the cool temperature against the summer heat wave we had been experiencing for over two record-breaking months.

Lying in the pitch darkness, I let my mind travel back in time over forty years spent with this man who was about to depart this old world. There had been both good times and bad, victories and defeats, times of laughter and despair. Blessings of three wonderful sons and seven precious grandchildren. Accomplishments and failures, all woven through with life lessons and growth. We were married much younger than we should have. Against all odds, we had made it, but only because of our shared faith in God.

I knew with certainty that without Him we would have become another statistic of a broken family and marriage. We had done the best we knew how to raise our kids to be responsible and good, and to carry on the legacy of our faith. Now, our time together was really ending, and it was too late to fix any unresolved problems or say anything left unsaid. I trusted God would continue to lead me through these next difficult hours and days as He had been so faithful to do since this season of my life had begun.

Peace washed over me as I again realized all He had done for us in the last twenty or so months of our lives. It had been astounding, really! I finally closed my weary eyes in complete security and safety, and sleep came quickly.

July thirtieth began as the previous few days had, with intense heat and stillness. As my two granddaughters moved about the house quietly, so as not to disturb Papa Jim, I showered quickly and began to prepare breakfast. In the evening, Chad and the girls left to go out to a family surprise birthday party which had been planned for several weeks.

Although Chad was reluctant to leave his dad's side, there had been no sign that Jim's condition had changed throughout the day. He and his wife Shana thought it might be good to get the girls out for a few hours to have fun and play with some of the other children who would attend the party.

Shana would stay at the house with me and planned to work on some classes she was taking online. I assured Chad if there was any change in Jim's condition, we would call him, and he could be back at the house in ten or fifteen minutes. After they left, Shana went to the computer in the spare bedroom, and I settled in on the couch by Jim's bed, taking a book to read with me.

About forty-five minutes later, Jim's breathing caught my attention, and I listened carefully for a couple of minutes. He had taken in long slow breaths, and then a few seconds passed before I heard another intake of air. This was exactly the transition the hospice worker had described.

I quickly called for Shana to come, and she was there in a flash beside me. We watched intently as Jim drew another long breath, followed by silence for a few seconds, then another long intake. The next space was much longer, and I took Shana's hand and said,

"Oh, Shana, is he going to be able to get another one?" I asked in panic.

"It's going to be okay," she said assuredly, as we both intently watched.

He finally breathed once again, but too much time had passed. This time, the seconds passed by one by one by one, but no breath came. As I went around the bed to draw close to him and take his hand, one single tear slid out of his right eye and traveled slowly down his face.

"Did you see that, Shana? I think he's telling us goodbye."

As it had all happened so quickly, it took me a moment to fully realize he was truly gone. I bent to give him one last kiss and whisper in his ear that I would see him again in heaven someday soon. God had spared him long hours of struggling to catch the next breath as the hospice worker had told me could happen. The last stage was mercifully brief, and God had taken him peacefully home.

Shana and I stood beside the bed and hugged each other for a long time, before she turned to go call Chad. I continued to stand at his bedside for a few lingering moments. Suddenly, God put one clear thought in my mind.

Cancer, you didn't win! God seized the victory, and in the blink of an eye, Jim was ushered into that magnificent, holy place of complete and miraculous healing.

What Cancer Cannot Do

Cancer is so limited.
YET IN ALL THINGS

It cannot cripple love, it cannot alter hope.
WE ARE MORE THAN CONQUERORS THROUGH HIM
WHO LOVED US

It cannot corrode faith, it cannot destroy peace.
I AM PERSUADED THAT NEITHER DEATH OR LIFE

It cannot kill friendship, it cannot suppress memories.
PRINCIPALITIES NOR POWERS, NOR THINGS PRESENT
NOR THINGS TO COME, NOR HEIGHT, NOR DEPTH

It cannot silence courage. It cannot invade the soul.
NOR ANY CREATED THING SHALL BE ABLE TO
SEPARATE
US FROM THE LOVE OF GOD

It cannot steal eternal life. It cannot conquer the spirit.
WHICH IS IN CHRIST JESUS OUR LORD

ROMANS 8:37-39

BARBARA RAMSEY

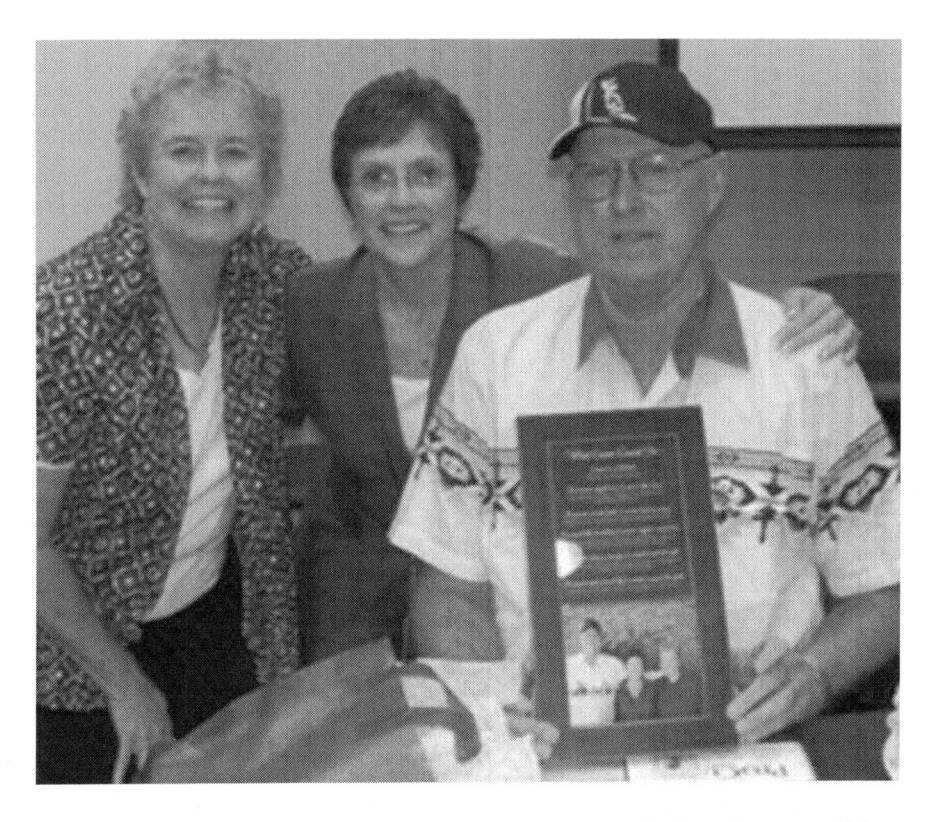

Barb, Peggy and Jim on Graduation Day with the plaque, *What Cancer Cannot Do*, given to Peggy.

This book can be ordered from Amazon and all on-line stores; it may be ordered from your local bookstore. If it has impacted your life for good, please share it with a friend or give it to your local library. Allow someone else to experience the miraculous provision, faith, love and hope of our great big God.

About 90% of all books sold are sold on Amazon. You can help spread the Word by sharing your impression of this book by giving a 'review' on Amazon.com. This is one of the best ways to help Barb in her ministry to help other people.

Made in the USA
San Bernardino, CA
22 March 2019